REFLEXIVITY

A Practical Guide for Researchers in Health and Social Sciences

REFLEXIVITY

A Practical Guide for Researchers in Health and Social Sciences

Edited by

Linda Finlay and Brendan Gough

Blackwell
Science

© 2003 by Blackwell Science Ltd
a Blackwell Publishing Company

Editorial offices:
Blackwell Science Ltd, 9600 Garsington Road, Oxford OX4 2DQ, UK
 Tel: +44 (0)1865 776868
Blackwell Publishing Inc., 350 Main Street, Malden, MA 02148-5020, USA
 Tel: +1 781 388 8250
Blackwell Science Asia Pty Ltd, 550 Swanston Street, Carlton, Victoria 3053, Australia
 Tel: +61 (0)3 8359 1011

First published 2003

Library of Congress Cataloging-in-Publication Data

Reflexivity: a practical guide for researchers in health and social sciences/edited by Linda Finlay and
 Brendan Gough.
  p. cm.
 Includes bibliographical references and index.
 ISBN 0-632-06414-5 (softcover)
 1. Social sciences–Research–Methodology. 2. Medical sciences–Research–Methodology.
 3. Qualitative research. 4. Reflection (Philosophy) I. Finlay, Linda, 1957– II. Gough, Brendan.

 H62.R3765 2003
 001.4′2–dc21
 2003051817

ISBN 0-632-06414-5

A catalogue record for this title is available from the British Library

Set in 10/13pt Sabon
by DP Photosetting, Aylesbury, Bucks.
Printed and bound in Great Britain using acid-free paper
by MPG Books Ltd, Bodmin, Cornwall

For further information on Blackwell Publishing, visit our website:
www.blackwellpublishing.com

Contents

Contributors

Linda Finlay PhD, BA(Hons), DipCOT, Consultant and Associate Lecturer, The Open University, Milton Keynes, UK

Brendan Gough PhD, BA(Hons), Lecturer in Qualitative Psychology, School of Psychology, University of Leeds, UK

Marla J. Arvay PhD, Associate Professor, Department of Educational and Counselling Psychology and Special Education, Faculty of Education, University of British Columbia, Canada

Claire Ballinger PhD, MSc, DipCOT, SROT, Lecturer in Occupational Therapy, School of Health Professions and Rehabilitation Sciences, University of Southampton, UK

Christine A. Barry PhD, BA, BSc, Research Fellow, Department of Human Sciences, Brunel University, UK

Gweneth Doane PhD, RN, Registered Psychologist, Associate Professor in the School of Nursing, Faculty of Human and Social Development, University of Victoria, Canada

Eugenie Georgaca PhD, MA, BA, Lecturer in Psychology, City College (affiliated to the University of Sheffield), Thessaloniki, Greece

David Harper PhD, BA(Hons), MClin Psychol, AFBPsS, Senior Lecturer in Clinical Psychology, School of Psychology, University of East London, UK

Katie MacMillan PhD, BSc, Research Associate, Business School, Loughborough University, UK

Ilja Maso PhD, MA(Hons), BA, Professor of the Theory of Science, University for Humanistics, Utrecht, The Netherlands

Alison McCamley MSc, BA(Hons), Senior Lecturer in Psychology, Department of Psychology, Sheffield Hallam University, UK

Majella McFadden PhD, BSc, Senior Lecturer, Department of Psychology, Sheffield Hallam University, UK

Elizabeth McKay PhD, SROT, ILTM, Head of Department of Occupational Therapy, School of Health Science, University of Limerick, Ireland

Paula Nicolson PhD, MSc, BSc, FBPsS, AcSS, Professor of Health Psychology, University of Sheffield, UK

Nick Rowe BA(Hons), RMN, SR Arts Therapist (Drama), Senior Lecturer, School of Professional Health Studies, York St. John College, UK

Susan Ryan MSc, BappSc, AccOT, SROT, OTR, Professor of Occupational Therapy, Department of Occupational Therapy, Faculty of Medicine and Health, University College, Cork, Ireland

Jonathan A. Smith, DPhil, MSc, BA, Senior Lecturer in Psychology, Birkbeck College, University of London, UK

Thelma Sumsion PhD, MEd, OT Reg(Ont), FCAOT, Director of the School of Occupational Therapy, University of Western Ontario, Canada

Prologue

'Reflexivity raises the most fundamental issue that can be raised for modern social enquiry' (Bonner, 2001, p.267).

Reflexivity in research seems, over the last decade, to have exploded into academic consciousness. Researchers, especially within the qualitative tradition, who are keen to acknowledge the situated nature of their research and to demonstrate the trustworthiness of their findings, are seeking new tools. Using reflexivity, they find that subjectivity in research can be transformed from problem to opportunity.

The etymological root of the word 'reflexive' means 'to bend back upon oneself'. In research terms this can be translated as thoughtful, self-aware analysis of the intersubjective dynamics between researcher and the researched. Reflexivity requires critical self-reflection of the ways in which researchers' social background, assumptions, positioning and behaviour impact on the research process.[1] It demands acknowledgement of how researchers (co-)construct their research findings. Reflexivity both challenges treasured research traditions and is challenging to apply in practice.

Beyond such definitions, we can also witness a 'confusing array of versions of reflexivity' – or 'reflexivities' (Lynch, 2000, p.27). For some, reflexivity is celebrated as part of our essential human capacity, while for others it is a self-critical lens. Some researchers utilise reflexivity to introspect, as a source of personal insight, while others employ it to interrogate the rhetoric underlying shared social discourses. Some treat it as a methodological tool to ensure 'truth', while others exploit it as a weapon to undermine truth-claims. Such diversity of uses makes it difficult both to understand the concept of reflexivity and to know how to apply it in practice.

---

[1] Reflection can be defined as 'thinking about' something after the event. Reflexivity, in contrast, involves a more immediate, dynamic and continuing self-awareness. We use the term critical self-reflection here in an attempt to capture both poles of the reflection–reflexivity continuum.

It is precisely this question of *how to do reflexivity in practice* that this book seeks to address. First and foremost, this book aims to be a *practical guide* to undertaking reflexive analysis at different stages of the research process. To this end we have invited eighteen authors (including ourselves) to share and critically examine their *versions of reflexivity*.

In Part I of the book, we (Linda Finlay and Brendan Gough) introduce the theoretical foundations and highlight some problematic issues concerning the practice of reflexivity. In Parts II–IV, the challenge of applying reflexivity in research practice is critically explored by the individual authors. Each chapter opens with a 'Biography Box' which situates the author's background and interests. Then they each tell their story, offering different versions of reflexivity – focused on personal, relational and collaborative elements respectively. (See the editorial introductions to each part.) The final chapter (Chapter 17) functions as the epilogue. With a flourish, Katie MacMillan offers a provocative and playful deconstruction of reflexive practices, challenging the conventional and the axiomatic.

As our authors reveal their dilemmas and struggles, we embrace their preparedness to be open and to keep asking questions. We continue to be impressed by the depth of their thoughtfulness, creativity and commitment to the reflexive project: their achievement far exceeds anything we could have done on our own. It was for this reason that we chose to produce an edited volume. We celebrate the *diversity* apparent across these contributions. The authors come from a range of backgrounds and countries and their disciplines span health care and social sciences. Beyond their various stances on reflexivity, the authors reveal differing theoretical and methodological commitments. Their chosen topics also vary: while some explore experiences of illness and health, others examine professional practice; while some focus on individual, personal journeys, others apply a wider lens, analysing social and political dimensions.

Of course, not every topic across the health care and social science fields could possibly be covered in just seventeen chapters. Certain voices are softer than others, and many are missing entirely. Yet we believe that the voices presented here reflect a broad range of reflexive practice and, as such, provide the basis for critical dialogue.

It remains for us to acknowledge our debts. Firstly, we are especially indebted to all the chapter authors for their support of this project. Distilling accounts of complex reflexive practices into just 5000 words was no mean feat. They rose to our challenge with enthusiasm and showed grace in the face of our shifting ideas. Secondly, we'd like to thank Sue Ram for her invaluable editing suggestions and her contribution in reviewing our final manuscript. Thirdly, our gratitude needs to be extended to Caroline Connelly, Commissioning Editor, Blackwell Publishing, both for believing in our project and for taking the manuscript on through publication.

Finally, we would like to share with you one particular challenge which arose during our project to produce this book on how to do reflexivity in practice. Each of us, authors and researchers, faced the inherent problem of providing a 'packaged account' of reflexivity when the process we experienced was considerably more confusing, complex, multi-layered, situational, tentative, emergent, precarious and messy than we could ever express. We have tried to guard against getting sucked into a vortex of narcissism, pretentiousness, or infinite regress, retaining, we hope, enough self-awareness to appreciate the ambiguous, slippery nature of our qualitative explorations. In this we have not always been successful. However, we ask you to tolerate the partiality of our understandings. At best, we can only offer you a glimpse into our research worlds. We leave the last word to Bourdieu, who elegantly expresses our position thus:

'The uncertainties and imprecisions of this deliberately foolhardy discourse thus have their counterpart in the quavering of the voice which is the mark of risks shared in any honest exchange of ideas and which, if it can still be heard, however faintly, through its written transcription, seems to me ... to justify its publication' (1990, p.ix).

Linda Finlay and Brendan Gough

References

Bonner, K.M. (2001) Reflexivity and interpretive sociology: the case of analysis and the problem of nihilism. *Human Sciences*, **24**, 293–325.

Bourdieu, P. (1990) *In Other Words: Essays Towards a Reflexive Sociology* (trans. Matthew Adamson). Polity Press, Cambridge.

Lynch, M. (2000) Against reflexivity as an academic virtue and source of privileged knowledge. *Theory, Culture & Society*, **17**(3), 26–54.

PART I

Introducing Reflexivity

For some commentators, reflexivity is a defining feature of human consciousness in a postmodern world. We are aware of being aware, of performing a variety of roles, and for some this implies that sincerity and authenticity have been replaced by irony and cynicism. Instead of imagining ourselves as coherent, unified beings, a postmodern sensibility compels us to recognise and celebrate diverse, shifting, and often contradictory self-fragments, to be playful and detached rather than engage seriously with questions about true or enduring values. Research into contemporary personhood, then, will mean an exploration of how people 'do' reflexivity in everyday life, how they construct and comment on multiple selves; in other words, an ethnomethodological project. But doing reflexivity should mean more than being clever and dispassionate – it should facilitate greater insights into personal and social experience. This is one of the reasons why some qualitative researchers have embraced reflexivity – it helps to situate the research project and enhance understanding of the topic under investigation. Reflexivity is a challenge to conventional ideals of science which favour professional distance and objectivity over engagement and subjectivity.

Reflexivity is also challenging to do. It requires huge efforts on the part of the researcher to identify and interrogate personal and professional practices. There is also some uncertainty and confusion about how reflexivity should be defined and practised – with examples of reflexivity poorly conceived and/or executed.

The main purpose of this introductory part of the book is to highlight important traditions and key debates pertaining to reflexivity. As Finlay points out in Chapter 1, reflexivity is a contested term. Different perspectives and methodological traditions exist, including humanistic-phenomenological and psychoanalytic emphasis on self-knowledge, 'critical' traditions such as feminism which prioritise socio-political positions, and social constructionist and 'postmodern' approaches which attend to discourse and rhetoric in the production of research texts. Finlay offers qualitative 'researcher-explorers' a map which identifies distinct variants of reflexivity. This typology of 'reflexivities' should help researchers decide which brands are most suitable for their particular research projects.

In Chapter 2, Gough addresses the critiques of reflexive qualitative research which have emerged within social constructionist, postmodern and discourse analytic work. For example, one strand of research has considered how some qualitative research has marshalled subjectivity as a means of authenticating research as more real, insightful or even 'objective', thereby reproducing the discourse of positivism which most qualitative researchers ostensibly reject. Attention to one's use of rhetorical devices can help militate against imagining a pure or 'true' account of the phenomenon in question. However, he argues that an undue preoccupation with language games can be distracting, even irritating, and that some balance needs to be struck between recognising the constructed nature of qualitative analysis and saying something coherent and relevant about the research topic itself. This chapter, then, opens up some thorny issues which reflexive researchers will need to negotiate without becoming embroiled in reflexive excess.

CHAPTER 1

The reflexive journey: mapping multiple routes

Linda Finlay

Positioning the self: author's story

Along with probably every other PhD student doing qualitative research, I struggled with questions relating to epistemology, ontology and methodology. In my phenomenological research on the life world of the occupational therapist I was a therapist studying other therapists. I wrestled with my role and position as researcher and academic. Challenged by the idea of relative perspectives, I grappled with my own subjectivity and struggled to evaluate its relevance to my research. Was it possible, or even desirable, for me to be 'objective'? If research is co-constituted, a joint product of participants, researcher and their relationship, how was I going to pin down something as abstract and ambiguous as 'intersubjective understandings'? How was I to represent a multiplicity of 'voices' while not hiding myself? Yet if I focused on myself as the producer of knowledge, wasn't there a risk that I would all too easily fall into the mire of the infinite regress, into excessive self-analysis and deconstructions? The problem seemed akin to being sunk in a 'swamp' (Finlay, 2002b).

Reflexivity became both my problem and my solution. My journey began, and with mounting excitement at discovering different dimensions of reflexivity, I explored and mapped different routes. I felt that I had first to understand the different ways of doing reflexivity before I could work out how to apply it to my specific research.

This chapter is the result – in a sense the map – of my intellectual struggle and journey. Here I identify at least five variants of reflexivity. The specific 'route' I eventually took in my own research – reflexivity as *hermeneutic reflection* – is described separately in Chapter 8.

Introduction: myriad forms of reflexivity

Reflexivity in qualitative research – where researchers turn a critical gaze towards themselves – has a history spanning at least a century. Moving from introspection towards critical realism, and then more recently towards postmodern deconstructionism, myriad forms of reflexivities have been practised. Although not always referred to explicitly as reflexivity, the *project of examining how the researcher and intersubjective elements impact on and transform research* has been an important part of the evolution of qualitative research. Critical self-reflective methodologies have evolved across different qualitative research fields in a story of shifts and turns.

Early anthropological 'realist tales', where researchers conscientiously recorded observations in an effort to prove their scientific credentials, have gradually given way to more personal accounts where researchers describe decisions and dilemmas of their fieldwork experience. Through the 1970s, a growing 'methodological self-consciousness' emerged. The ethnographic critique of ethnography (led by writers such as Clifford & Marcus, 1986[1]), pushed qualitative researchers into a 'new paradigm, placing discovery of reflexivity at the centre of methodological thinking' (Seale, 1999, p.160).

In highly subjectivist accounts of fieldwork, ethnographers and anthropologists (among other qualitative researchers) were concerned to unravel how their biographies intersect with their interpretation of field experiences. These fieldworkers portrayed themselves as infiltrating a group and then reporting on their experiences as an 'insider'. Other researchers, on a more 'objective' mission, sought to increase the validity and trustworthiness of their findings. They used reflexivity to continually monitor and audit the research process. They sought to transform personal experience into public (and so accountable) knowledge:

'Transactions and the ideas that emerge from [the research process] ... should be documented. The construction of analytic or methodological memoranda and working papers, and the consequent explication of working hypotheses, are of vital importance. It is important that the processes of exploration and abduction be documented and retrievable' (Coffey & Atkinson, 1996, p.191).

In these ways a research history is offered as both a confessional tale (Van Maanen, 1988) and a transparent account of the research. The practice of offering better ('truer'?) methodological accounts towards affirming the validity of research, however, was itself challenged as regretful backward glances at positivist ideals. Instead, postmodern researchers sought a more radical reflexivity as they embraced the negotiated, relative and socially constructed nature of the research experience. In an explicit and particular critique of earlier imperialist and colonialist anthropologies (for example, Clifford & Marcus, 1986, docu-

---

[1] This edited collection entitled *Writing culture: the poetics and politics of ethnography* marked a turning point in the anthropological literature. The authors moved towards a postmodern stance which shed doubt that any method, theory or tradition had a privileged claim to authoritative knowledge. Increasingly 'truth claims' were suspected as serving particular (political) interests.

mented the complicity of researchers in the story of colonialism), they attempted to erode the researcher's privileged position. A new 'self–other' consciousness – where the boundaries between the researcher and the researched is blurred – came to the fore.

Feminist versions of reflexivity (for example, Wilkinson, 1988 and Reinharz, 1992) also emerged at this time to address concerns about unexamined power balances between participants and researchers. Hertz, for instance, urges researchers to be aware of their own positions and interests and to explicitly situate themselves within the research. She argues that researchers are 'imposed at all stages of the research process – from the questions they ask to those they ignore, from who they study to who they ignore, from problem formulation to analysis, representation and writing – in order to produce less distorted accounts of the social world' (1997, p.viii).

Today, 'narratives of the self' proliferate. The growing body of reflexive and narrative research on the experience of disability is a case in point (Frank, 1998; Toombs, 2001). Also, in works such as Kondo (1990) reflexive feminism and cultural critique converge (Marcus, 1994). At the same time the sociological, post-structuralist turn in writings abounds as researchers concentrate on the discursive and macro-sociopolitical forces shaping research narratives. 'Self-reflexivity unmasks complex political/ideological agendas hidden in our writing' (Richardson, 1994, p.523). The researcher 'appears not as an individual creative scholar, a knowing subject who discovers, but more as a material body through whom a narrative structure unfolds' (Bruner, 1986, p.150).

The last couple of decades have also seen a surge of interest in writing processes and innovative styles. Writers (for instance, Geertz, 1988) now favour less authoritative and more self-critical texts which explicitly acknowledge that research findings are partial, partisan and fundamentally anchored in the social context. Self-reflexive experimental writing forms (for instance Tyler, 1987 and Ashmore, 1989), replete with parody, irony and scepticism, are favoured as being more in tune with our postmodern world. Creative and evocative representations are also seen to enable researchers to relate differently to their material.

Reflexivity in all its guises is now, arguably, a defining feature of qualitative research (Banister et al., 1994). As qualitative researchers, we now accept that the researcher is a central figure who actively constructs the collection, selection and interpretation of data. We appreciate that research is co-constituted – a joint product of the participants, researcher and their relationship. We realise that meanings are negotiated within particular social contexts so that another researcher will unfold a different story. We no longer seek to abolish the researcher's presence – instead, 'subjectivity in research is transformed from a problem to an opportunity' (Finlay, 2002a, p.531). In short, researchers no longer question the need for reflexivity: the question is *how to do it?*. The debate inhabits the space between researchers of different theoretical persuasions who lay claim to competing accounts of the rationale and practices of reflexivity.

In this introductory chapter, I look at how researchers from a range of research traditions have undertaken their reflexive journey, drawing on examples from their research. I offer a typology ('maps') of what seems to be occurring in contemporary practice. Five variants of reflexivity are explored: (1) introspection, (2) intersubjective reflection, (3) mutual collaboration, (4) social critique and (5) ironic deconstruction (see also Finlay, 2002b for a fuller account). This way of conceptualising reflexivity[2] shows how routes vary according to researchers' aims and focus. As with any typology, the borders overlap and could well be drawn differently. These limitations notwithstanding, it seems important to distinguish between different variants of reflexive research in practice.

Each variant of reflexivity carries its own strengths and weaknesses; each presents particular opportunities and challenges. I hope that the maps offered will enable us as 'researcher-explorers' to make a deliberate and informed choice of route as we embark on our own reflexive journeys.

Reflexivity as introspection

When Maslow (1966) asserted 'there is no substitute for experience, none at all' (1966, p. 45), he pointed researchers towards the value of self-dialogue and discovery. Those researchers who begin their research with the data of their experience seek to 'embrace their own humanness as the basis for psychological understanding' (Walsh, 1995, p.335). Here, the researcher's own reflecting, intuiting and thinking are used as primary evidence (Moustakas, 1994).

Moustakas (1990) describes this process in terms of forming the research question: 'The task of the initial engagement is to discover an intense interest, a passionate concern that calls out to the researcher' (1990, p.27). Moustakas' phenomenological work on loneliness, for instance, began at a critical time in his life when he was faced with a problem of whether or not to agree to major heart surgery that might restore his daughter to health or result in her death. 'The urgency of making a critical decision plunged me into the experience of feeling utterly alone ... I became aware that at the center of my world was a deep and pervasive feeling of loneliness' (1990, p.91).

---

[2] Numerous typologies have, of course, been published. Lynch (2000) offers an inventory of 'reflexivities': mechanical, substantive, methodological, meta-theoretical, interpretative and ethnomethological. Two particular notable, and often referenced, typologies are the ones by Marcus (1994) and Wilkinson (1988). Marcus (1994) identifies four 'styles' of reflexivity: (1) self-critique and personal quest, (2) objective reflexivity as a methodological tool, (3) reflexivity as 'politics of location' and (4) feminist experiential reflexivity as the practice of 'positioning' (of standpoint epistemologies). Wilkinson (1988) offers her feminist distinction between personal (i.e. subjective factors), functional (as related to one's researcher role) and disciplinary (looking at the place and function of the particular research project) reflexivity.

In his personal, anthropological account of how being paralysed resulted in his loss of self, Murphy (1987) discloses the following:

'From the time my tumor was first diagnosed through my entry into wheelchair life, I had an increasing apprehension that I had lost much more than the full use of my legs. I had also lost a part of my self. It was not just that people acted differently toward me, which they did, but rather that I felt differently toward myself. I had changed in my own mind, in my self-image, and in the basic conditions of my existence. It left me feeling alone and isolated ... it was a change for the worse, a diminution of everything I used to be' (Murphy, 1987, p.85).

Beyond probing personal experience and meanings for their own sake, such introspection can yield insights which then form the basis of a more generalised understanding and interpretation. Self-reflections are assumed to provide data regarding the social/emotional world of participants. As Parker (1997, p.488) reminds us, 'We need to be aware of ourselves as the dreamers ... unlike instances of other people telling us their dreams, we understand and share, partially at least, at some level, the story.'

A powerful example of this comes from Rosaldo (1993) in his influential anthropological study of Ilongot head-hunting. Here he drew on his personal experience of bereavement (the death of his wife) to make sense of the rage the men felt which pushed them to head-hunt. Similarly, Abu-Lughod's experience of learning to live as a 'modest daughter' within a Bedouin community offers an example of how generating experiential data can contribute to a broader analysis – in this instance of women's modesty and veiling practices:

'It was at this moment, when I felt naked before an Arab elder because I could not veil, that I understood viscerally that women veil not because anyone tells them to or because they would be punished if they did not, but because they feel extremely uncomfortable in the presence of certain categories of men' (Abu-Lughod, 1988, cited in Hertz, 1997, p.98).

The use of personal experience is also picked up by psychodynamic researchers who explore how unconscious fantasies can be mobilised in research encounters. Kracke's (1987, cited in Hunt, 1989) anthropological work with South American Indians provides a good illustration. Here, competition with father images and castration anxieties became important themes. Noting how the tribe openly expressed feelings and fantasies normally disguised in Western cultures, Kracke was confronted by his own fantasy life:

'Even now, in intense periods of working though conflicts, I find myself practically redreaming the dreams that were told to me by Jovenil or Francisco [his participants] – if not literally in the manifest content of my own dreams, at least taking a very important place in the latent content. I am sure at some level I was seeking something like this when I chose to work with South American Indians in the first place . . . But the point here is the degree to which the experience was integrated into my personality – through my transference to Jovenil and . . . others' (cited in Hunt, 1989, pp.32–3).

Ultimately, reflexivity should be 'neither an opportunity to wallow in subjectivity nor permission to engage in legitimised emoting' (Finlay, 1998, p.455). The challenge for researchers using introspection is to use personal revelation not as an end in itself but as a springboard for interpretations and more general insight. In this sense, the researcher moves beyond 'benign introspection' (Woolgar, 1989, p.22) to become more explicit about the link between knowledge claims, personal experiences of both participant and researcher, and the social context. This message carries through into the second variant of reflexivity which argues against individual and 'inner' subjectivity dislocated from the intersubjective research relations.

Reflexivity as intersubjective reflection

The genre of reflexivity as intersubjective reflection has grown significantly in the past decade and can be found across a range of phenomenological, feminist, psychoanalytical and ethnographic research. Here, researchers explore the mutual meanings involved within the research relationship. They focus on the situated, emergent and negotiated nature of the research encounter and, for those of a psychodynamic persuasion, how unconscious processes structure relations between the researcher and participant. The process here involves more than reflection – instead, a radical self-reflective consciousness (Sartre, 1969) is sought where the self-in-relation-to-others becomes both the aim and object of focus. Moreover, in psychodynamic terms, 'construing both researcher and researched as anxious, defended subjects', Hollway (2001, p.15) reminds us 'that both will be subject to projections and introjections'. These dynamics can become the focus for analysis.

Researchers employing this variant of reflexivity commonly turn a critical gaze towards the emotional investment they have in the research relationships concerned. In their research on subjectivity and crime Hollway and Jefferson (2000) utilised reflexivity along with their narrative method using psychoanalytic interpretations. Jefferson, for example, describes his sense of rapport and identification with Tommy, one of their participants:

'A big reason for this good rapport, I felt, stemmed from our both being members of big families. He never knew that about me, but listening to him talking about his family produced points of identification which to some extent bridged our class, educational and work differences, probably enabling me to be a better, more informed listener. His clean, tidy, well-kept house (unlike some we entered), his active involvement in community affairs, including running a local kids' football team ... facilitated my identification with him ... In short, I enjoyed interviewing Tommy because I liked him; and I liked him because we had things in common.'

Jefferson goes on to describe how he used his subjective feelings along with theory to probe his participant's account:

'Our theoretical starting-point was undoubtedly important in alerting us to the contradictory nature of Tommy's account, but so too was my subjective feeling on reading it; how disjunctive it felt to my experience ... It might be objected that my memories are no more reliable than Tommy's and that I am projecting on to him my own feelings about unpleasant aspects of my childhood. This possibility can be tested against Tommy's text ... Our judgement is that they are present in the detail but shorn of the emotion which would naturally accompany them. It is that accompaniment that I feel I know and can use empathically here' (2000, pp. 65–6).

Scott (1995, cited in Johnson & Scott, 1997) studied 17 families as they moved through the child protection system. She writes of the strong emotional reactions aroused in her which came as a surprise as she was an experienced practitioner. As a researcher, she felt a sense of helplessness witnessing the distress which she could not alleviate, plus an unease with the inherent voyeurism of research observations:

'What caused me the most anguish was not the abuse itself, but witnessing children and their parents who appeared to me to be suffering at the hands of professionals ... The professionals were seemingly unaware of the pain their actions had inflicted ... This led to me developing a strong identification with the vulnerability of clients and a deepening ambivalence towards members of my own profession ... My thesis supervisor observed the censorious tone which was sometimes audible in the "authorial voice" in my field notes. ...'

Scott goes on to note how her emotional reactions provided interesting insights into the phenomena being explored:

'[The] negative feelings ... being aroused in me ... led me to see in a new way the hostility I observed being expressed between different professions and organisations toward one another ... Interagency conflict in child protection cases [would seem to be] related to displacement of hostility' (Johnson & Scott, 1997, pp.35–7).

In this vein, psychodynamic researchers remind us to explore how conversation or text affects us and to reflect on what we bring to it ourselves. In particular, they see unconscious needs and transferences as mutually structuring the relationship between researcher and participant. 'The inner worlds of researchers', Hunt (1989) notes, 'structure their choice of setting, experience in the initial stages of fieldwork, and the research roles they assume. The transferences that are situationally mobilised in the fieldwork encounter have implications for the questions researchers ask, the answers they hear, and the materials they observe.' 'Most important', she continues, 'transferences structure the researcher's ability to develop empathic relations with those subjects who provide the essential source of sociological data' (1989, p.81).

In her work on the police, Hunt (1989) identifies how her status as an unwanted female outsider raised a number of issues (of which she had been unconscious) which then impacted on her research relationships:

'Positive oedipal wishes also appeared to be mobilized in the fieldwork encounter. The resultant anxieties were increased because of the proportion of men to women in the police organization and the way in which policemen sexualized so many encounters... The fact that I knew more about their work world than their wives also may have heightened anxiety because it implied closeness to subjects. By partly defeminizing myself through the adoption of a liminal gender role, I avoided a conflictual oedipal victory. That the police represented forbidden objects of sexual desire was revealed in dreams and slips of the tongue ... the intended sentence "Jim's a good cop" came out instead "Jim's a good cock." In those words, I revealed my sexual interest in a category of men who were forbidden as a result of their status as research subjects. In that way, they resembled incestuous objects' (p.40).

Examples such as these highlight the value of examining the research relationship. This project is not without challenges, however. The difficulties of gaining access to personal (and possibly unconscious) motivations should not be underestimated, while the complex dynamics between inter-*acting* researcher and participant add a further layer of opacity. To accomplish such a feat, it could be argued, requires a 'superhuman self-consciousness' attainable only through intensive psychoanalysis (Seale, 1999). Countering these challenges, researchers interested in exploring intersubjective dynamics defend their mission to explore the co-constituted nature of the research looking both inward for personal meanings and outward into the realm of shared meanings, interaction and discourse. These themes also provide the focus for researchers interested in collaborative enquiry.

Reflexivity as mutual collaboration

Researchers making use of reflexivity as mutual collaboration are found using a broad range of methodologies, from humanistic new paradigm and co-operative inquiry research (e.g. Heron, 1996; Reason, 1988) to more sociological, discursive and feminist research approaches (e.g. Wilkinson, 1988; Banister *et al.*, 1994; Potter & Wetherell, 1995; Yardley, 1997). These wide-ranging research methodologies are linked by the way they seek to enlist participants as co-researchers and vice versa.

Recognising research as a co-constituted account, adherents of participative research argue that research participants also have the capacity to be reflexive beings. they can be co-opted into the research as co-researchers. At the very least this involves participants in a reflexive dialogue during data analysis or evaluation.

Co-operative inquiry approaches, on the other hand, apply reflexivity more completely. Here researchers, simultaneously participants in their own research, engage in cycles of mutual reflection and experience. A fascinating reflexive study of interactive interviewing by Ellis *et al.* (1997, p.121) provides insights into how a research relationship develops and shapes the findings produced. In this exploration of the researchers' experience of bulimia, they describe their work as 'sharing personal and social experiences of both respondents and researchers, who tell ... their stories in the context of a developing relationship':

> 'Lisa and I are masters at intellectualizing bulimia. Through our conversations, I have moved beyond a literal interpretation of bulimia as being only about thinness to thinking about how eating disorders also speak to personal longings. But, it always has been hard for us to focus on emotional issues. I have come to see this as a relational problem to which we both contribute ... Bulimia is about mess. Lisa and I talk about it, study it, analyze it, and WE DO IT! As perfectionists ... we craft exteriors that contradict the mess in our lives. Still I know what goes on "behind the closed doors" in Lisa's life, because I know what goes on behind my own closed doors' (1997, pp.127–8).

Drawing on research by Traylen (1994) into the role of health visitors, Heron (1996) describes a co-operative inquiry where the co-researchers/co-participants engage in a reflexive dialogue about their research process:

> 'Just when we were feeling so confident the group was thrown into confusion, uncertainty and depression ... We were swamped by the enormity of the task and scared about whether we would be able to make sense of it all ... The group's pre-occupation with action had, I think, something to do with avoiding the key issue of our lack of clarity about the health visitor's role, which had always been present hovering in the wings. I had no idea how were going to address this. All I could hang onto at this stage was the thought that if the group could hold this chaos for long enough perhaps something would emerge' (cited in Heron, 1996, p.149).

While these studies are to be valued for their collaborative, democratic, inclusive spirit, critics reject the pronounced element of compromise and negotiation which could potentially 'water down' the insights of single researchers. In reply, collaborative researchers argue that dialogue within a group allows members to move beyond their preconceived theories and subjective understandings towards representing multiple voices. Halling (1999), makes this point in his discussion on a dialogic, phenomenological study on forgiveness he carried out in collaboration with a group of Masters students:

> 'Working in dialogue and comparing personal experiences and the interviews with each other allowed us to come to a rich, collective understanding of the process of forgiving another... Freedom infuses the process with a spirit of exploration and discovery, and is evident through the group members' ability to be playful and imaginative with their interpretations. Trust provides the capacity to be genuinely receptive to what is new and different in the others' experiences and expressions and accounts for respect toward each person's descriptions, interpretations, and stories' (1999, p.11).

Collaborative reflexivity offers the opportunity to hear, and take into account, multiple voices and conflicting positions. While the notion of shared realities finds favour with many researchers, some still challenge an egalitarian rhetoric where it disguises essentially unequal relationships. It is this last issue which is taken up in the fourth variant of reflexivity.

Reflexivity as social critique

Johnson and Scott (1997) examine the way their two ethnographic studies (on deinstitutionalisation of women and on child protection practices respectively) sought to 'provide a voice for the unheard' and how, as researchers, they 'identified strongly with the people who were subject to the power of others' (1997, p.40). Exemplifying reflexivity as social critique, they go on to highlight some problematic and coercive institutional practices.

One particular concern for researchers using reflexivity as social critique is how to manage the power imbalance between researcher and participant. They openly acknowledge tensions arising from different social positions, for instance, in relation to class, gender and race. As Wasserfall (1997) explains, 'the use of reflexivity during fieldwork can mute the distance and alienation built into conventional notions of "objectivity" or objectifying those who are studied. The research process becomes more mutual, as a strategy to deconstruct the author's authority' (1997, p.152).

Reflecting retrospectively, Willott (1998) examines the individual, sociopolitical and research implications of being a feminist researcher researching men:

'There is a tension between being a researcher and being a feminist. As a feminist I want to see a change in the patriarchal relations between men and women. I would like this change to extend to my relationships with the research participants, but found it difficult to challenge directly. As a researcher I was careful to nurture relationships, to avoid stepping over invisible lines in which these relationships might be jeopardized, and to "enter sympathetically into the alien and possibly repugnant perspectives of rival thinkers"' (1998, p.183).

In their feminist account of researching 'Asian' women's experience of child-birth, Marshall *et al.* (1998, p.128) probe how they were centrally implicated in the representation of their research participants. In particular, they acknowledge how this involved some selective silence on their part when it came to writing up their research:

'We have used accounts ... to point to care where the woman is viewed and treated on the basis of ethnic grouping ... But additionally, in these extracts there is a singling out of black nurses. This raises the issue of what to do when working with marginalized accounts which themselves reproduce prejudicial viewpoints and evaluations. Our decision to date has been not to report these aspects of the accounts. (Leaving silenced aspects of the accounts that we do not want to hear?) ... These tensions around the representation of "experience" were and are central for us as researchers. In adjudicating between what and what not to write up we could be accused of taking the political-moral highground ... this sort of "suppression" results in a misunderstanding of power ... and hence, prevents opportunities for countering oppression which currently exist.'

Burns (2002) offers the following social constructionist analysis where she explores issues around her own embodiment which emerged while interviewing participants who binge eat and use vomiting, laxatives, exercising and fasting to compensate:

'Lisa's initial uninvited appraisal of my body ... as "slim" elicited a feeling of power, comfort and relief, followed quickly by a sense of shame and guilt. When I reflected on this exchange I remembered feeling simultaneously happy and uncomfortable with her admiring assessment that I was con-forming to certain standards of femininity. This demonstrates the impor-tance of acknowledging and accepting that the bodies of the researcher and participant are both subject to interpretation and production through cul-tural discourses. ... During one moment when large bodies were being described in derogatory terms I remember this producing a feeling of "fat-ness", being greedy and guilt due to the large lunch I had eaten just prior to the interview ... I momentarily wished I had not eaten so much and resolved to go running later that day to "make up" for my indulgence. Reflecting critically about this reaction resulted in an appreciation of the effects of discourses of slenderness at the level of my own embodied subjectivity. I was interpellated in a physical way by the discourses articulated by the woman I was speaking with.'

Reflexivity as social critique offers the opportunity to utilise experiential accounts while situating these within a strong theoretical framework about the social construction of power. A particular strength with this account is the recognition of multiple, shifting researcher–participant positions. The task of deconstructing the author's authority, however, carries associated costs. As with the previous variant, preoccupations with egalitarianism can divert attention away from other, possibly more pertinent, issues and can result, paradoxically, in a strategy which lays claim to more authority. Such rhetorical strategies are the focus of the final variant of reflexivity.

Reflexivity as ironic deconstruction

Reflexivity as ironic deconstruction, in common with some versions of reflexivity as social critique, arises out of a postmodern, post-structuralist paradigm. This perspective sees the world as a babble of competing voices, none of which has privileged status. In this view, the researcher's imperative is to challenge and unravel the rhetoric of being a 'voice of authority' enabling, instead, multiple voices to be heard.

In reflexivity as ironic deconstruction, attention is paid to the ambiguity of meanings in language used and to how this impacts on modes of presentation. How, researchers ask, can we pin down and represent the dynamic, multiple meanings embedded in language? Woolgar (1989) suggests one route forward is to juxtapose 'textual elements such that no single (comfortable) interpretation is readily available. In this scheme, different elements manifest a self-referring or even contradictory relation with one another' (1989, p.85). In his thesis on 'Wrighting sociology of scientific knowledge' – a classic example of ironic reflexivity – Ashmore plays upon and parodies the circumstances of the pro-duction of his doctoral thesis by interspersing entertaining, fictional dialogues with literature reviews and dialectical critique:

'It is not enough to take reflexivity as one's topic . . . It sets out to be a mode of inquiry. The self-destructive solution of noninquiry in which paradoxical problems are outlawed, and only the others suffer, is no solution at all. Indeed, by showing and displaying and talking around its own socially constituted nature, its own textuality and its own paradox, instead of always and only talking *of* these things, it can talk of other things . . . Celebratory practical reflexive inquiry is wrighting beyond the tu quoque. And it must be shown, not told' (Ashmore, 1989, p.110).

This variant of reflexivity follows through its radical project by refusing to exempt the sociology of science from its own scrutiny. 'Rather than attempting to evade paradoxes created by applying relativist arguments to themselves', Lynch (2000, p.37) notes, 'they celebrate paradox and argue that it is threatening only to those who hold on to a restricted and outmoded conception [of] certainty and logical compulsion'.

Researchers inclined towards social constructionism focus more explicitly on deconstructing the language used and its rhetorical functions (see Billig *et al.*, 1988). 'Factual and fictional stories share many of the same kinds of textual devices for constructing credible descriptions, building plausible or unusual event sequences, attending to causes and consequences, agency and blame, character and circumstance', explains Edwards (1997, p.232). Researchers from this tradition would notice how both participants and researchers are engaged in an exercise of 'presenting' themselves to each other – and to the wider community which is to receive the research.

Other postmodern researchers have focused on reflexive writing itself in terms of textual radicalism. Lincoln and Denzin (1994) explain how textual experimentation reflects a move towards a postmodern pluralism, which qualitative research needs to reflect. Here, there is 'not one "voice", but polyvocality; not one story but many talks, dramas, pieces of fiction, fables, memories, histories, autobiographies, poems and other texts' (1994, p.584). In such a spirit, Harvey (2002), utilised poetry in order to represent the ambiguity and multiplicity of meaning that seemed to be at the core of what he was encountering in his research on organisations, managers and their employees:

'Here One Minute...'

Go for it!	not coping
Capture the moment!	live the lie
Be strong!	keep schtum
Take no prisoners!	bite tongue
Do the business!	doing just enough
Prove yourself!	as become pissed off
Prioritise!	distressed
Manage it!	deskilled
Be empowered!	delayered
Feel the Fear!	gone.

Harvey goes on to explain how the poem better captures the 'starkness and bluntness' of his participant's delivery and the 'raw emotion of his talk of the culture he found himself part of (and colluding with)'. Through the poem Harvey was able to avoid sanitising the research encounter and his own reactions.

Irony and creative evocative presentations can be thought-provoking and may help to balance any authorial claims. At the same time there is a risk that self-conscious, 'clever' presentations are taken so far that they can alienate, become pretentious or even lose all meaning. Postmodern researchers employing reflexivity to deconstruct objective claims have the paradoxical problem of the status of their own project.

Opportunities and challenges

Reflexivity, then, can be understood in a multitude of ways according to the aims and functions of the exercise at stake and the theoretical or methodological traditions embraced. In terms of aims, reflexivity can be understood as a confessional account of methodology or as examining our own personal, possibly unconscious, reactions. It can mean exploring the dynamics of our researcher–researched relationship. Alternatively, it can focus more on how the research is co-constituted and socially situated, through offering a critique or through deconstructing pretences of established meanings. The functions of reflexivity shift from employing it to offer an account of the research to situating the researcher and voicing difference; from using reflexivity to interpret and understand in terms of data analysis to attending to broader political dimensions when presenting material.

In terms of theoretical and methodological commitments, the 'social critique' and 'ironic deconstruction' variants favoured by postmodernists, social constructionists and sociologists stand in opposition to the more personal and individual stance of 'introspective' phenomenological and psychodynamic researchers. At the same time, feminists and other socially minded researchers would embrace several of the variants valuing both the experiential and critical dimensions. The attention paid to critical, relativist values in some variants offers a stark contrast to the realist intentions of some essentialist or methodologically focused accounts. The style adopted in 'intersubjective reflection' can be more descriptive (as with phenomenological accounts) or explanatory, when psychodynamic interpretations come into play. Decisions about which variant of reflexivity to embrace need to take into account these different epistemological values and assumptions.

Taking reflexivity as a whole, in its various guises, we can see that it has the potential to be a valuable tool, as something that can help us:

- Examine the impact of the position, perspective and presence of the researcher.
- Promote rich insight through examining personal responses and interpersonal dynamics.
- Open up unconscious motivations and implicit biases in the researcher's approach.
- Empower others by opening up a more radical consciousness.
- Evaluate the research process, method and outcomes.

● Enable public scrutiny of the integrity of the research through offering a methodological log of research decisions (Finlay, 2002a, p.532).

However, as we have also seen, reflexivity is not without its critics or its pitfalls. In offering a methodological account, researchers seeking to promote the integrity of the research need to grapple with the problematic spectre of having a single, 'true' account. Does the process of explicitly situating the researcher invariably produce a better account or might it function as an unwitting strategy to claim more authority? When researchers focus on their own experiences, as in the case of reflexive 'introspection', may not the researcher's voice eventually overshadow that of the participant? In the case of reflexivity as 'intersubjective reflection' and mutual 'collaboration' (assuming it is even possible to unravel such complex dynamics), focusing on the interpersonal process may shift attention away from the phenomena being studied. In a different way, researchers using reflexivity to deconstruct or as 'social critique' have to grapple with shifting subject positions and slippery meanings as they strive to find a balance between profitable deconstruction and nihilism.

So which is the best route for reflexivity? Surely the more pertinent question is *how well we do our reflexive analysis?* Introspection and intersubjective reflection without critical self-analysis is surely of limited value and open to the charge of self-indulgence. Collaborative reflexivity which fails to reveal conflicting voices and lacks a well-grounded critical rationale can rhetorically disguise inequalities present. In the case of reflexivity as social critique, it is naive, if not disingenuous, to pay lip-service to the power dimension by assuming a fixed and knowable subject position: the focus, instead, needs to be on the diverse and shifting positions mutually adopted. Finally ironic deconstructions, taken too far, can become irritating rather than thought-provoking. Ultimately, 'what reflexivity does, what it threatens to expose, what it reveals and who it empowers depends upon who does it and how they go about it' (Lynch, 2000, p.36).

It is the task of each researcher, based on our research aims, values and the logic of the methodology involved, to decide how best to exploit the reflexive potential of our research. Each of us will choose our road. For all the difficulties inherent in the task, to avoid reflexive analysis altogether is likely to compromise the research. 'It would be fundamentally incomplete', says Bonner (2001, p.273), for social researchers '*not* to make reflexivity an essential component of social analysis.'

Summary

This chapter has mapped the routes taken by different researchers who have laid claim to competing, sometimes contradictory, accounts of the rationale and practice of reflexivity. Each way of approaching reflexivity carries opportunities and costs, has strengths and limitations. The challenge – whichever the mode of reflexivity embraced – is to do the reflexive analysis well. And so the journey begins. . . .

Acknowledgement

With kind permission from Sage Publications Ltd, this chapter has been reprinted substantially from Finlay, L. (2002) Negotiating the swamp: the opportunity and challenge of reflexivity in research practice. *Qualitative Research*, **2**(2), 209–30.

References

Ashmore, M. (1989) *The Reflexive Thesis: Wrighting Sociology of Scientific Knowledge.* The University of Chicago Press, Chicago.

Banister, P., Burman, E., Parker, I., Taylor, M., & Tindall, C. (1994) *Qualitative Methods in Psychology: A Research Guide.* Open University Press, Buckingham.

Billig, M., Condor, S., Edwards, D., Gane, M., Middleton, D. & Radley, A. (1988) *Ideological Dilemmas: A Social Psychology of Everyday Thinking.* Sage Publications, London.

Bonner, K.M. (2001) Reflexivity and interpretive sociology: the case of analysis and the problem of nihilism. *Human Studies*, **24**, 267–92.

Bruner, E.M. (1986) Ethnography as narrative. In *The Anthropology of Experience* (Turner, V. & Bruner, E., eds). University of Illinois Press, Chicago.

Burns, M. (2002) Interviewing: embodied communication. Paper given at *International Human Sciences Research Conference*, Victoria, Canada.

Clifford, J. & Marcus, C.E. (eds) (1986) *Writing Culture: The Poetics and Politics of Ethnography.* University of California Press, Berkeley.

Coffey, A. & Atkinson, P. (1996) *Making Sense of Qualitative Data Analysis: Complementary Strategies.* Sage Publications, Thousand Oaks, CA.

Edwards, D. (1997) *Discourse and Cognition.* Sage Publications, London.

Ellis, C., Kiesinger, C.E. & Tillmann-Healy, L.M. (1997) Interactive interviewing: talking about emotional experience. In *Reflexivity and Voice* (Hertz, R., ed.). Sage Publications, Thousand Oaks, CA.

Finlay, L. (1998) Reflexivity: an essential component for all research? *British Journal of Occupational Therapy*, **61**, 453–6.

Finlay, L. (2002a) 'Outing' the researcher: the provenance, principles and practice of reflexivity. *Qualitative Health Research*, **12**(3), 531–45.

Finlay, L. (2002b) Negotiating the swamp: the opportunity and challenge of reflexivity in research practice. *Qualitative Research*, **2**(2), 209–30.

Frank, A.W. (1998) Just listening: narrative and deep illness. *Families, Systems & Health*, **16**(3), 197–212.

Geertz, C. (1988) *Works and Lives: The Anthropologist as Author.* Stanford University Press, Stanford, CA.

Halling, S. (1999) Dialogal research: a 'gritty' approach to phenomenological practice. Paper presented at *Symposium on Phenomenological Research*, Perugia, Italy.

Harvey, B. (2002) Encountering empowerment rhetoric: conjunctions and disjunctions of managers and the managed. PhD thesis, University of Leicester.

Heron, J. (1996) *Co-operative Inquiry: Research into the Human Condition*. Sage Publications, London.

Hertz, R. (Ed.) (1997) *Reflexivity and Voice*. Sage Publications, Thousand Oaks, CA.

Hollway, W. (2001) The psycho-social subject in 'evidence-based practice'. *Journal of Social Work Practice*, **15**(1), 9–22.

Hollway, W. & Jefferson, T. (2000) *Doing Qualitative Research Differently: Free Association, Narrative and the Interview Method*. Sage Publications, London.

Hunt, J.C. (1989) Psychoanalytic aspects of fieldwork. *Qualitative Research Methods Volume 18*. Sage, Newbury Park.

Johnson, K. & Scott, D. (1997) Confessional tales: an exploration of the self and other in two ethnographies. *The Australian Journal of Social Research*, **4**(1), 27–48.

Kondo, D. (1990) *Crafting Selves: Power, Gender and Discourses of Identity in a Japanese Workplace*. University of Chicago Press, Chicago.

Lincoln, Y.S. & Denzin, N.K. (1994) The fifth movement. In *Handbook of Qualitative Research* (Denzin, N.K. & Lincoln, Y.S., eds). Sage Publications, Thousand Oaks, CA.

Lynch, M. (2000) Against reflexivity as an academic virtue and source of privileged knowledge. *Theory, Culture & Society*, **17**(3), 26–54.

Marcus, G.E. (1994) What comes (just) after 'Post'?: the case of ethnography. In *Handbook of Qualitative Research* (Denzin, N.K. & Lincoln, Y.S., eds). Sage Publications, Thousand Oaks, CA.

Marshall, H., Woollett, A. & Dosanjh, N. (1998) Researching marginalized standpoints: some tensions around plural standpoints and diverse 'experiences'. In *Standpoints and Differences* (Henwood, K., Griffin, C. & Phoenix, A., eds). Sage Publications, London.

Maslow, A.H. (1966) *The Psychology of Science*. Harper and Row, New York.

Moustakas, C. (1990) *Heuristic Research: Design, Methodology and Applications*. Sage Publications, Newbury Park, CA.

Moustakas, C. (1994) *Phenomenological Research Methods*. Sage Publications, Thousand Oaks, CA.

Murphy, R. (1987) *The Body Silent*. Henry Holt, New York.

Parker, I. (1997) Discourse analysis and psychoanalysis. *British Journal of Social Psychology*, **36**, 479–95.

Potter, J. & Wetherell, M. (1995) Discourse analysis. In *Rethinking Methods in Psychology* (Smith, J.A., Harre, R. & Van Langenhove, L., eds). Sage Publications, London.

Reason, P. (ed.) (1988) *Human Inquiry in Action*. Sage Publications, London.

Reinharz, S. (1992) *Feminist Methods in Social Research*. Oxford University Press, New York.

Reinharz, S. (1997) Who am I? The need for a variety of selves in the field. In *Reflexivity and Voice* (Hertz, R., ed.). Sage Publications, Thousand Oaks, CA.

Richardson, L. (1994) Writing: a method of inquiry. In *Handbook of Qualitative Research* (Denzin, N.K. & Lincoln, Y.S., eds). Sage Publications, Thousand Oaks, CA.

Rosaldo, R. (1989) *Culture and Truth: Renewing the Anthropologist's Search for Meaning*. Beacon, Boston.

Rosaldo, R. (1993) Introduction: grief and a headhunter's rage. In *Culture and Truth: The Remaking of Social Analysis* (Rosaldo, R., ed.). Routledge, London.

Sartre, J. (1969) *Being and Nothingness*. Routledge, London.

Seale, C. (1999) *The Quality of Qualitative Research*. Sage Publications, London.

Toombs, S.K. (2001) Reflections on bodily change: the lived experience of disability. In *Phenomenology and Medicine* (Toombs, S.K., ed.). Kluwer Academic Publishers, Dordrecht, Holland.

Tyler, S.A. (1987) *The Unspeakable: Discourse, Dialogue, and Rhetoric in the Postmodern World*. University of Wisconsin Press, Madison.

Van Maanen, L. (1988) *Tales of the Field: On Writing Ethnography*. University of Chicago Press, Chicago.

Walsh, R.A. (1995) The approach of the human science researcher: implications for the practice of qualitative research. *The Humanistic Psychologist*, **23**, 333–44.

Wasserfall, R.R. (1997) Reflexivity, feminism and difference. In *Reflexivity and Voice* (Hertz, R., ed.). Sage Publications, Thousand Oaks, CA.

Wilkinson, S. (1988) The role of reflexivity in feminist psychology. *Women's Studies International Forum*, **11**, 493–502.

Willott, S. (1998) An outsider within: a feminist doing research with men. In *Standpoints and Differences* (Henwood, K., Griffin, C. & Phoenix, A., eds). Sage Publications, London.

Woolgar, S. (1989) Foreword. In *The Reflexive Thesis: Wrighting Sociology of Scientific Knowledge* (Ashmore, M.). The University of Chicago Press, Chicago.

Yardley, L. (Ed.) (1997) *Material Discourse of Health and Illness*. Routledge, London.

CHAPTER 2

Deconstructing reflexivity

Brendan Gough

Positioning the self: author's story

As a qualitative researcher and social psychologist, my work has been heavily shaped by social constructionist and (more recently) psychoanalytic thinking. I am enlightened by the way social constructionism helps explain how individuals are inserted into society, and I am also convinced by psychoanalytic accounts of (inter-)subjective affiliations and motivations. In terms of analysing qualitative data, I have drawn upon discourse analytic approaches (see Potter & Wetherell, 1987; Burman & Parker, 1993) and am also turning to modes of data collection and interpretation informed by psychoanalytic theory (see Hollway & Jefferson, 2000). Although both traditions espouse very different conceptual repertoires, social constructionism and psychoanalysis converge in presenting the subject as defined by forces largely beyond control, whether they be prevailing discourse(s) or unconscious identifications. As such, a radical challenge is posed to humanistic (and Western) themes of agency, choice, responsibility – and reflexivity. How can an individual know which societal and unconscious forces prompted particular courses of action? Similarly, how can a researcher identify subjective influences on the research process?

Postmodern responses to this problem have stressed multiple researcher and participant voices, and some have turned to poetic and dramatic forms of writing to highlight complexity in subjectivity and representation generally (e.g. Denzin, 2001). Others, influenced by ethnomethodology and conversation analysis, have concentrated on enactments of reflexivity as topics for study (see Lynch, 2000). In this chapter, I argue that both these positions are overly preoccupied with style over substance and end up avoiding issues of responsibility for and ownership of the research. I suggest that qualitative researchers should attempt a balance between flat, unreflexive analyses and excessive, hyper-reflexive analyses. In this way, something can be said about the topic under investigation, as well as how this understanding was constructed.

Introduction

In this chapter I proceed from the first chapter in presenting reflexivity as multi-faceted and the subject of much debate in contemporary social science. In this light I argue for the plural term 'reflexivities' in order to move away from the notion that reflexivity is something that can be captured once and for all, something that we can all agree upon. In the section on 'Doing reflexivity' I then suggest that opportunities to practise whatever brand of reflexivity can be limited by established writing and publishing conventions. The next section critiques realist forms of reflexivity, arguing that these can serve as a means of privileging the analyst's account, of reinforcing a supposedly accurate or 'true' interpretation of the phenomenon. I then consider postmodern variants on reflexivity which concentrate on language games and often deploy techniques from art and literature to deconstruct authorship. I also reflect on ethnomethodological treatments of reflexivity which study how reflexivity is warranted by researchers and laypeople alike. Both these postmodern and the ethnomethodological approaches to reflexivity are problematic in over-prioritising language use at the expense of coherent analysis of researcher subjectivity and the research topic. Finally, some balance between the extremes of realism and textual radicalism is advocated, emphasising the importance of reflexivity, but not to the extent that the analyst and the phenomenon disappear from view.

Reflexivities

For qualitative researchers, reflexivity facilitates a critical attitude towards locating the impact of research(er) context and subjectivity on project design, data collection, data analysis, and presentation of findings. It refers to a set of practices which help distinguish qualitative from quantitative forms of inquiry (where the emphasis is on the suppression of material pertaining to the process of research, including researcher subjectivity) and which facilitates insights into the context, relationships and power dynamics germane to the research setting (Wilkinson, 1988). As such, the personal is celebrated as a strength by qualitative researchers, a resource to be exploited in order to enrich the quality of analysis (Finlay, 2002).

Reflexivity is signalled by the researcher's incorporation of information relating to the research context and to relevant personal thoughts and feelings into the research report. But there is great variation in practice. Reflexivity may be concentrated at one stage of the research, or applied throughout the research process. It may be enhanced through discussion with colleagues and/or research participants, or simply by regular solitary reflections recorded in a research journal or diary. As Finlay notes in the previous chapter, diverse definitions of and theoretical positions on reflexivity will inform how different qualitative researchers practise reflexivity. Clearly, research informed by psychoanalysis will approach reflexivity differently from humanistic work or social constructionist projects. Some of the debates between distinct perspectives will be touched on in this chapter, particularly regarding the functions of reflexive accounts and the status of researcher knowledge. Because of this lack of consensus concerning the conception and application of reflexivity, I want to endorse the term reflexivities (Lynch, 2000; Pels, 2000) to signify current plurality, flexibility, and conflict.

Several researchers have attempted to summarise different positions on, and practices of, reflexivity and in so doing have effectively captured complexities (see Marcus, 1994; Lynch, 2000; Finlay, 2002). By way of highlighting diversity and setting the scene for the ensuing deconstruction of reflexivity, I now draw upon an early, much cited paper by Wilkinson (1988) which identifies three distinct but interrelated forms of reflexivity: *personal*, *functional* and *disciplinary*.

At the very least, reflexivity implies that the researchers make visible their individuality and its effects on the research process. There is an attempt to highlight those motivations, interests and attitudes which the researcher has imported to the research and to reflect on how these have impacted on each stage. Such subjective factors are typically construed as bias or interference within 'scientific' research, but recognition of the personal dimension to research is heralded as enriching and informative by qualitative researchers. For example, researchers conducting an interview study on experiences of parenthood might fruitfully reflect on their motivations for choosing such a topic (to better understand their experiences of parenthood or being parented; to gather knowledge on a phenomenon which they themselves are considering), their choice of interview questions (a focus on family/work balance), interviewees (of similar age to themselves) and their expectations about what the research might yield (a view of parenthood as challenging, fulfilling or isolating). Such self-awareness can help inform data collection. For example, if the researcher has experience of parenthood, a stance of respect and empathy relating to the interviewees could be used to develop a rich understanding of this phenomenon. When collecting data, personal thoughts and feelings prompted by the interviews/interviewees should be recorded – it is likely that experiences with different people will produce diverse reactions. Data analysis can then be informed by the researcher's data as well as that of the participants.

But reflexivity extends beyond the personal domain. Wilkinson's (1988) second variant, 'functional reflexivity', relates to one's role as a researcher and the effects this might have on the research process. It focuses attention on the different identities presented within the research and the interactions between researcher and participants. Here, a key issue concerns the distribution of power and status within the research process. Although many qualitative researchers are committed to democratic forms of inquiry where the voices of participants are encouraged and respected, it is virtually impossible to escape researcher–participant relationships structured by inequalities (see Parker, 1992). After all, it is the researcher who generally develops an idea, formulates the research questions and organises the format of the research. For many qualitative researchers, such taken-for-granted ideas and professional routines should be destabilised as far as possible (Taylor & White, 2000). In my own work on men and masculinities, I draw attention to the subject positions and power relations which pertain to the research context, which mostly favour the researcher (e.g. as expert interrogator) but which at times indicate participant status and researcher vulnerability, as when participants suddenly depart from the script and direct difficult questions to the researcher (see Chapter 11).

Wilkinson's (1988) third category, 'disciplinary reflexivity', involves a critical stance towards the place and function of the particular research project within broader debates about theory and method. It suggests delineating those existing concepts and traditions which have been important in shaping the research and calls for some discussion of the potential contribution of the research to a particular literature. This political dimension of reflexivity is enthusiastically endorsed by feminist and critical researchers interested in challenging the findings of conventional (usually quantitative) social science research (see Stainton-Rogers et al., 1995). For example, work by Gill (1993) on indirect sexism challenges psychological and liberal humanist values which construct prejudice as individual pathology rather than social practice promoted by dominant institutions and reproduced in everyday talk. In her critical analysis of sexist talk, the aims of (social) psychological research are rewritten to address the oppression of marginalised groups rather than simply reflecting prevailing social norms (see Gough & McFadden, 2001 for an introduction to 'Critical Social Psychology').

Doing reflexivity

Reflexivity, then, can mean many things, and perhaps works best when different forms or levels are recognised and practised. Reflexivity which dwells only on one level may appear impoverished. An exclusive focus on personal reflexivity, for example, does not situate research within relevant interpersonal, institutional and cultural contexts, and as a result the analysis may seem unduly limited. But how do ideas about reflexivity translate into practice? In this section, I provide a brief account of popular reflexive practices, before proceeding to interrogate the way reflexivity has been enacted within certain traditions of qualitative research.

One useful preliminary strategy is to look at one's choice of research question(s), and how this question is framed. It is often helpful to arrange for a colleague to assume the role of devil's advocate, challenging one's chosen research plan and perhaps tentatively suggesting alternatives. As a result, one might end up with better research questions, and some insight into personal motivations and values. Maso (this volume) proposes using the 'why interview' ('why this, why not that?') as a means to clarify and refine one's research interests, whereby the researcher's plans are placed under the spotlight until a more satisfactory version emerges. I think one would need to be careful here to ensure an egalitarian exchange of views, as a critique of one's original ideas might prove disheartening for inexperienced researchers. But if handled well, explicating and revising one's research goals can prove extremely enlightening and set the scene for a more rewarding research experience.

As a general rule, reflexivity implies rendering explicit hidden agendas and half-formed intentions, but not just at the start of the research process – this should be a continuous endeavour. Many qualitative researchers favour some form of research diary or journal which documents the researcher's thoughts and experiences before, during and after data collection and analysis (Banister *et al.*, 1994). Notes concerning why certain choices and decisions were made, about changing directions, personal reactions etc. can be used to inform a 'reflexive account' which in turn will inform the research report. Again, asking oneself difficult questions can facilitate enhanced reflexivity and, ultimately, greater understanding of the phenomenon under investigation. In research projects involving other members, issues raised in one's research diary can be brought back to the team for discussion. Of course, team members may well offer differing, even conflicting, perspectives on a given matter, and this process would need to be carefully managed (see Barry, this volume).

Another interesting approach is to promote reflexivity in participants, in parallel to that being practised by the researcher(s). Of course, participant reflexivity is implicitly encouraged by certain methodologies, such as diary studies, where reflection on social interactions and personal relationships might be encouraged. Co-operative inquiry approaches may ask participants to consider data previously gathered and analysed to stimulate thinking about, say, continuities and changes in the transition from pregnancy to motherhood (see Smith, this volume). This practice clearly goes beyond the common strategy of offering one's data analysis to participants for their commentary in order to help validate researcher interpretations. On the other hand, facilitating participant reflexivity throughout the project would be a significant feature of collaborative and action research projects where there is a concerted effort to reduce power differentials between researcher and researched, to establish a team of equal status co-researchers (e.g. Reason, 1988; Banister *et al.*, 1994). Feminist researchers, for example, might tackle the subordination of women at a particular site (a workplace, a leisure facility) by enlisting local women as active participants in conceiving, designing and enacting the research plan (see Rheinharz, 1992).

In practising reflexivity, it is often useful to articulate a theoretical position which can help stimulate critical thinking (see Finlay, 2002). A phenomenological commitment, for example, would prompt sustained self-reflection in order to reveal personal values and intersubjective experience relevant to the phenomenon in question (see Giorgi, 1985). Indeed, anecdotal evidence suggests that researchers often have a vested interest in studying specific topics in the first place, so any insight into such personal investments might prove valuable. In contrast, a social constructionist orientation would entail locating the researcher within prevailing discourses pertaining to, say, gender and work, if the research was on the meaning(s) of unemployment. Here, identifying the subject positions available to the researcher (and others) would help illuminate the social construction of unemployment.

It is my own personal view that concepts and strategies from psychoanalytic theory can fruitfully inform research reflections and reflexivity generally. I find it a little strange that discussions of reflexivity rarely make reference to psychoanalytic theory, despite a long and rich tradition of writing on intersubjective dynamics. Of course psychoanalytic writing has attracted widespread critique from a variety of perspectives, much of it well-justified, but I agree with Frosh (1997) when he contends that there are valuable concepts which can be drawn upon by social scientists in making sense of materials. The concept of countertransference may be especially useful as a way for researchers to gain access to their unanticipated (unconscious) thoughts and feelings pertaining to specific research encounters. Better understanding of the case in question may well ensue (see also Hollway & Jefferson, 2000).

Theoretical predilection notwithstanding, the incorporation of one's reflections into the analysis and writing-up process is a vexed issue, with many authors preferring simply to provide information about researcher and participant subject positions (gender, age, social class, race etc.) and perhaps hazarding some speculation towards the end of the paper on the effects of these factors on the research outcomes. This limited, undergraduate form of reflexive accounting is perhaps encouraged by established journals which prioritise the reporting of results within tight word limits (see Kleinman, 1991) and ensures that more substantial reflexive analyses are mainly confined to unpublished writing (e.g. doctoral theses) or more specialist texts (such as this volume). This is an issue which I feel needs to be addressed within the community of qualitative researchers. While I do not advocate limitless space to muse about research processes and intersubjective encounters, I believe the conventions for inscribing qualitative research within recognised journals and books need to be revised to facilitate analyses which are properly interrogated and contextualised.

Reflexivity and realism

At another level, the functions of reflexive writing need to be examined, since what may pass as reflexivity may, upon scrutiny, draw upon the idioms of quantitative research. Being 'open' about researcher subjectivity and its impact on the research process sounds like a good idea, but the presumption of access to subjective feelings and values has been radically challenged in the wake of the linguistic turn in social theory heralded by postmodernism, social construction-ism and discourse analysis (see Kvale, 1992; Gergen, 1991; Potter & Wetherell, 1987). The notion that reflexive researchers can uncover their 'real' motivations if they dig deep enough is reminiscent of the discourse of positivism which argues that the 'truth' about the objective world can be revealed through rigorous application of scientific methods. Researcher honesty or openness may be imagined, but because neither the researcher nor anyone else can ever establish 'true' intentions or motivations, then such claims must be treated with suspicion. In this section I consider the implications of social constructionism for under-standing the presentation of research and look at some of the discursive strategies used by qualitative researchers to render their analyses objective. I go on to argue that reflexive attention to our discourse(s) as researchers can help prevent a preoccupation with positivist ideals of objectivity and can enable a more vibrant form of writing.

If we take seriously social constructionist and/or postmodern perspectives on subjectivity, which conceptualise the subject as decentred, fragmented, relational, evolving and incomplete (see Kvale, 1992; Wetherell & Maybin, 1996), then the notion of uncovering underlying personal influences becomes problematic. Denzin (2001, p.28) notes: '... there is no essential self or private, real self. There are only different selves, different performances, different ways of being a gen-dered person in a social situation.' (It is also worth pointing out that, historically, psychoanalytic theory highlighted this problem of subjective awareness, arguing that what we know about ourselves is but a defensive fiction which obscures our 'real', irrational and confused self).

Social constructionism (e.g. Burr, 1995) and discursive psychology (e.g. Edwards & Potter, 1992) contest the notion that language/interpretation reflects reality, arguing, on the contrary, that interpretations – even those given by 'authoritative' sources such as scientists and doctors – construct reality. For example, work on the sociology of scientific knowledge (SSK) has drawn atten-tion to an 'empiricist repertoire' which scientists, including psychologists, use to bring off a depersonalised account of the 'facts' (e.g. Woolgar, 1980). An obvious demonstration of this repertoire is the use of the passive voice ('the experiment was conducted', rather than 'I conducted the experiment'). When authorship *is* acknowledged, the collective, institutional 'we' is preferred. Such 'externalising devices' are also witnessed in other contexts, such as journalism ('the facts state that...'; 'the evidence suggests...') (Gilbert & Mulkay, 1984). Other work on doctor–patient communication has identified further strategies for legitimating professional accounts, such as 'category entitlement', which refer to the use of categories (e.g. doctor–patient) in talk which mobilise culturally prescribed expectations about who is knowledgeable. For example, when the term 'doctor' is used in conversation it commonly denotes status and expertise and can be used to warrant certain accounts and to challenge those of patients, 'laypeople' or others (see Silverman, 1987).

But qualitative researchers are not immune from using rhetorical devices to convey the authenticity of their analyses, whether reflexive or not. In contrast to suppressing the (human) processes of data collection and analysis as a means of legitimating accounts, qualitative researchers have achieved the same goal through recognising, even celebrating, personal input into the research endeavour. Such reflexive accounting, which draws attention to researcher as well as participant practices, constructs the researcher as expert witness, immersed in or close to the scene or phenomenon under investigation. Seale (1999) locates this form of accounting within anthropological writing, whereby researcher entry into other groups or cultures is presented as an ideal vantage point for better observations. Such confessions are often told in great depth (detail is a way of enhancing credibility) and suggest an invaluable, objective insider account. In this sense, reflexivity can be used to warrant data analysis as truthful or rich, thereby falling back on positivist notions of objectivity (but, ironically, through subjectivity).

In fact, instances of allegiance to realist epistemology abound in the literature on qualitative research. For example, Hall and Callery (2001) have recently argued that reflexivity should be used by grounded theorists in order to improve rigour. It is widely felt that such endeavours can enhance the transparency, accountability and general trustworthiness of qualitative research (see Coffey & Atkinson, 1996). More broadly, there is a major emphasis on validating analytic claims via a range of techniques, such as member checking, audit trail and triangulation (see Denzin & Lincoln, 1994). Clearly, the discourse structuring these activities is one of truth-seeking, a quest for an interpretation to which all parties can subscribe.

Seale (1999) refers to a study by Buckingham *et al.* (1976) of wards for terminally ill patients to illustrate the point. In Buckingham *et al.*'s research account, emphasis is placed on the great lengths that the researcher went to in order to gain insight into ward life – the researcher subjected himself to various physical invasions to pass as a credible candidate for admission to the hospital. Once inside the ward as a 'patient', he recorded his observations from this valued position and later included them in published reports in order to validate the analysis about regimes of care on the ward.

So, even when a positivist view of research is critiqued (as is often the case in papers which proceed to endorse the use of qualitative methods), writers can end up (unwittingly) reproducing a positivist discourse which prioritises rigour and accuracy. Discourse analysts have produced a considerable literature on how speakers and writers, including researchers, work to construct accounts as persuasive and legitimate. It is argued that greater awareness of the assumptions and practices habitually deployed in research and professional discourse generally can aid greater reflexivity, what White (1997) calls 'epistemic reflexivity'. For example, credibility of the speaker or writer is frequently carried off through 'stake inoculation' (Potter, 1996) whereby personal interest ('stake') is disavowed to suggest that the 'facts' are independent. Typically, ground is prepared to position the speaker outside the event or situation, as a rational detached observer (much like the stance of the scientist within the empiricist repertoire). Consider the practice of suspending presuppositions which is popular in some phenomenological research and forms of grounded theory so that a (pure) focus on data is enabled and, ultimately, an analysis which is more objective, less contaminated, can result.

Another strategy used in the reporting of research is to set up a 'contrast structure' (Smith, 1978) whereby one element (e.g. established 'quantitative' research) is presented in a negative light which then enables another element (e.g. your 'qualitative' research) to come across as superior. Positive aspects of the subordinated element may even be admitted ('some research in this tradition has produced interesting findings, but...') before one's own contribution is presented as distinctive and progressive, albeit perhaps modestly ('In contrast to previous research, what I hope to show is...').

One must also bear in mind the degree of editing and selectivity which informs the process of writing up such 'insider' analyses, say for submission to an academic journal. Only pre-specified aspects of researcher involvement may be presented to an academic audience, perhaps to highlight the researcher's credentials in conducting the research (e.g. self-identifying as a 'feminist' in studies of gender), whilst others might be omitted (e.g. instances of discomfort in the research process, such as questions which don't work or moments of researcher defensiveness, although these could also be included, coded as initial shortcomings in a narrative of progress culminating in the 'truth'). Pressures towards offering a coherent narrative aligned with more prosaic constraints such as word limits will inevitably mean that contradictions are glossed over and only a small selection of categories and data extracts are included in the finished paper.

Qualitative researchers interested in doing reflexivity then, need to attend to their discourse, the rhetoric used to produce accounts of researcher involvement, the research process and analysis of the phenomenon. Indeed, researchers influenced by postmodernism and related approaches have attempted to demonstrate awareness of researcher and other voices in order to de-privilege and de-stabilise conventional understandings of authorship. This 'meta-reflexivity' is evident in experimental writing whereby established formats for social scientific presentation are undermined, although such endeavours raise complex issues, as we shall see.

Reflexivity as deconstruction

Metaphors for describing contemporary or postmodern society tend to emphasise pluralism, such as 'polyvocality' (Lincoln & Denzin, 1994) and 'saturation' (Gergen, 1991). These metaphors have informed how some qualitative research gets reported. One technique is to disrupt the narrative flow of the text with commentaries at the end of each section, thereby counter-posing the academic analysis with more personal (e.g. identifying researcher emotions) reporting (Lather, 1992). In this way, the dual positions of the researcher become apparent and some self-doubt might be intimated by the researcher (e.g. Rosaldo, 1993), although the personal may still be used to warrant interpretations as superior to traditional, distanced investigations (Seale, 1999).

But some qualitative researchers have gone further, advocating a more radical disruption of narrative conventions concerning coherence and representation. Some have striven to make the author/analyst disappear altogether by simply presenting participant's data with minimal or no commentary (e.g. Dwyer, 1982), although one wonders about processes of selection and editing which produce an apparently pure text (Seale, 1999).

Avoiding interpretation strikes me as somewhat pointless, and seems to rely on a realist repertoire where the data somehow 'speaks for itself'. Others have turned to the creative arts for inspiration and have rendered qualitative analyses in the form of poetry (e.g. Richardson, 1994), dramatic dialogue (e.g. Paget, 1995), narrative collage and montage (Dillard, 1982). According to one definition, 'performative writing' is 'evocative, reflexive, multi-voiced, criss-crosses genres, is always partial and incomplete' (Pollock, 1998, cited in Denzin, 2001). The deployment of fictional forms and characters fundamentally disarms claims about authenticity and authorship, and arguably enlivens scientific writing. This postmodern reflexivity evokes rather than represents (Tyler, 1987).

However, concerns have been raised about such innovative literary-minded texts. Sometimes they can come across as rather self-indulgent and narcissistic, as if analysts are attempting to realise hitherto frustrated desires to become artists. Also, the de-centring of the author in such accounts often masks decision-making processes in the production of the account, i.e. authorship. Questions about how data extracts were selected and reworked remain. Despite claims about opening up social scientific writing towards more egalitarian formats comprising multiple voices, invariably the analyst plays a dominant role in writing and editing the 'script'. According to Law (1994, p.190): '... literary devices abound and self-referential loops relieve readers of the burden of engagement for, in reading these accounts, they appear "strangely self-contained, sealing themselves off from comment and criticism"' (cited in May, 1999, p. 32). In ethnography, Murphy (2002) has lamented the pre-eminence of style over substance and worries that the discipline may 'implode under its own inward gaze' (p.259). Similarly, in discussing some examples from the postmodern genre, Seale (1999, p.176) argues that the author should be reinstated and that transparency in accounting procedures should remain paramount: 'Although powerful in their ability to convey particular meanings, fictional and dramatic forms should be used with caution by researchers in case they discourage authors from making clear presentations of the evidence that has led to particular conclusions'.

Another strand of research deriving from ethnomethodology and conversation analysis subjects reflexive discourse itself to analysis. Within this tradition, reflexive activities become the topic, the data to be examined (e.g. Lynch, 2000; Slack, 2000). Here, questions about and commitments to specific forms of reflexivity and what constitutes good qualitative research are sidestepped in favour of analysing how reflexivity is claimed and enacted. After all, contemporary social theorists have pointed out that we are all reflexive now, that we live in a reflexive society and so forth, so that reflexivity is not just confined to qualitative research, but is a mundane activity which permeates selfhood and relationships today (Giddens, 1984). In other words, there is nothing special about reflexivity conducted by academics – 'ordinary' people do reflexivity, and the ways they do it should be the subject of social scientific investigation, as opposed to social scientists using reflexivity to produce more interesting, provocative or relevant analyses.

But an exclusive focus on 'member's' accounting procedures as advocated by ethnomethodology and conversation analysis implies that the researcher is detached from the researched – no presuppositions are admitted or interrogated (May, 1999). It is as if scrupulous descriptions of everyday language use absolve the researcher from taking up positions vis-à-vis positioning in the social world, i.e. within societal discourses which define and constrain speakers according to gender, race, sexual orientation etc. According to Atkinson (1988, p.446), 'the radical stress on observable details risks becoming an unprincipled, descriptive recapitulation devoid of significance . . . minute descriptive detail is assembled in a hyper-realist profusion, until the reader loses any sense of meaning' (cited in May, 2000).

Whilst careful attention to participant's language is important, I believe that qualitative researchers should not shy away from making pronouncements which situate this language within wider social and cultural currents. Ethnomethodology has presented an important critique of scholarly overinterpretation, but it would be a mistake to throw out the baby of standpoint with the bathwater of representation. In other words, researchers should take responsibility for making intelligible interpretations rather than exclusively concentrating on participant's accounts (or opting for fictional presentations). But researcher involvement should be examined critically, reflexively, so that analysis is not overdetermined. A balance is required between opening and closure, between deconstruction and reconstruction, between recognising our qualitative analyses as constructed (and perhaps using some devices from art and literature to deconstruct our analysis), and – temporarily at least – settling for a version of analysis with which we are satisfied, which we think makes a valid theoretical and/or political point (see Latour, 1988).

Recovering reflexivity

In sum, some balance between the extremes of unreflexive, 'flat' description, which presents a supposedly 'objective' picture of the phenomenon, and convoluted, meta-reflexive textual presentations, which move too far away from the phenomenon in question, is recommended. This is what Pels (2000) calls 'one-step up' reflexivity: 'a self-conscious exercise in circular reasoning, which breaks with the unending quest for a transcendent objectivity, and rests satisfied with merely partial and partisan perspectives' (p.15). More succinctly, Pels notes that 'it is both feasible and important to talk about something and simultaneously talk (at least a little) about the talking itself' (p.3).

Other theorists use different terminology and advocate slightly different 'solutions': Harding (1991) prefers 'strong reflexivity' over conventional ('weak') objectivity, while Bourdieu (1981) advocates 'scientific' reflexivity over 'narcissistic' or 'nihilistic' reflexivity. This balance can be seen in some feminist and critical psychological appropriations of discourse analysis (e.g. Parker, 1992: 'critical realism'; Gill, 1993: 'politically informed relativism') which argue against relativism in order to hold on to a standpoint (for example women as oppressed within discourses of motherhood) for political and practical purposes. Indeed, various efforts have been made within feminism to move beyond both modernist confidence and postmodern nihilism towards a position which doesn't prescribe inertia, variously termed 'fractured foundationalism' (Stanley & Wise, 1993), 'interactive universalism' (Benhabib, 1992) and 'strategic essentialism' (Grosz, 1990).

Summary

To conclude, reflexivity is a contested term, attracting diverse definitions and associated with a range of activities and goals. A broad distinction can be made between *realist* uses of reflexivity, wherein researcher confession is deployed to reinforce the 'accuracy' or 'authenticity' of analysis, and postmodern or *relativist* forms of reflexivity, which tend towards disrupting narrative coherence and advertise analysis as constructed. I have argued that neither version of reflexivity is exclusively desirable, that researchers need to take some responsibility for producing an analysis which can be applied to support a particular view of the world, whilst recognising researcher involvement in the production of the account. In the chapters which follow, there are several examples of qualitative researchers doing just that, and offering good advice for practising and enhancing reflexivity in the process.

References

Atkinson, P. (1988) Ethnomethodology: a critical review. *Annual Review of Sociology*, **14**, 441–65. Cited in May, T. (2000) Reflexivity in social life and sociological practice: a rejoinder to Roger Slack. *Sociological Research Online*, 5(1), http://socresonline.org.uk/5/1/may.html

Banister, P., Burman., E., Parker, I., Taylor, M. & Tindall, C. (1994) *Qualitative Methods in Psychology: A Research Guide*. Open University Press, Buckingham.

Benhabib, S. (1992) *Situating the Self: Gender, Community and Postmodernism in Contemporary Ethics*. Polity, Cambridge.

Bourdieu, P. (1991) The specificity of the scientific field. In *Sociology: Rupture and Renewal Since 1968* (Lemert, C.C., ed.). Columbia University Press, New York.

Buckingham, R.W., Lack, S.A., Mount, B.M., Maclean, L.D. & Collins, J.T. (1976) Living with the dying: use of the technique of participant observation. *Health Education Quarterly*, **19**, 117–35.

Burman, E. & Parker, I. (1993) *Discourse Analytic Research. Repertoires and Readings of Text in Action*. Routledge, London.

Burr, V. (1995) *An Introduction to Social Constructionism*. Routledge, London.

Coffey, A. & Atkinson, P. (1996) *Making Sense of Qualitative Data Analysis: Complementary Strategies*. Sage Publications, Thousand Oaks, CA.

Denzin, N. (2001) The reflexive interview and a performative social science. *Qualitative Research*, 1(1), 23–46.

Denzin, N.K. & Lincoln, Y. (1994) *Handbook of Qualitative Research*. Sage Publications,, Thousand Oaks, CA.

Dillard, A. (1982) *Living by Fiction*. Harper & Row, New York.

Dwyer, K. (1982) *Moroccan Dialogues: Anthropology in Question*. Johns Hopkins University Press, Baltimore, MD.

Edwards, D. & Potter, J. (1992) *Discursive Psychology*. Sage Publications, London.

Finlay, L. (2002) Negotiating the swamp: the opportunity and challenge of reflexivity in research practice. *Qualitative Research*, **2**, 209–30.

Frosh, S. (1997) *For and Against Psychoanalysis*. Routledge, London.

Gergen, K. (1991) *The Saturated Self: Dilemmas of Identity in Contemporary Life*. Basic Books, New York.

Giddens, A. (1984) *The Constitution of Society: Outline of the Theory of Structuration*. Polity, Cambridge.

Gilbert, G.N. & Mulkay, M.J. (1984) *Opening Pandora's Box: A Sociological Analysis of Scientists' Discourse*. Cambridge University Press, Cambridge.

Gill, R. (1993) Justifying injustice: broadcaster's accounts of inequality. In *Discourse Analytic Research: Repertoires and Readings of Texts in Action* (Burman, E. & Parker, I., eds). Routledge, London.

Giorgi, A. (1985) *Phenomenology and Psychological Research*. Duquesne University Press, Pittsburgh.

Gough, B. & McFadden, M. (2001) *Critical Social Psychology: An Introduction*. Palgrave, London.

Grosz, E. (1990) A note on essentialism and difference. In *Feminist Knowledge: Critique and Construct* (Gunew, S., ed.). Routledge, London.

Hall, W.A. & Callery, P. (2001) Enhancing the rigor of Grounded Theory: incorporating Reflexivity and Relationality. *Qualitative Health Research*, **11**(2), 257–52.

Harding, S. (1991) *Whose Science? Whose Knowledge?* Open University Press, Buckingham.

Hollway, W. & Jefferson, T. (2000) *Doing Qualitative Research Differently: Free Association, Narrative and the Interview Method.* Sage Publications, London.

Kleinman, S. (1991) Field-workers' feelings: what we feel, who we are, how we analyse. In *Experiencing Fieldwork: An Inside View of Qualitative Research* (Shaffir, W.B. & Stebbins, R.A., eds). Sage, Newbury Park, CA.

Kvale, S. (ed.) (1992) *Psychology and Postmodernism.* Sage Publications, London.

Lather, P. (1992) Postmodernism and the human sciences. In *Psychology & Postmodernism* (Kvale, S., ed.). Sage Publications, London.

Latour, B. (1988) The politics of explanation: an alternative. In *Knowledge and Reflexivity: New Frontiers in the Sociology of Knowledge* (Woolgar, S., ed.). Sage Publications, London.

Law, J. (1994) *Organising Modernity.* Basil Blackwell, Oxford.

Lincoln, Y.S. and Denzin, N.K. (1994) The fifth movement. In *Handbook of Qualitative Research* (Denzin, N. & Lincoln, Y., eds). Sage Publications, Thousand Oaks, CA.

Lynch, M. (2000) Against reflexivity as an academic virtue and source of privilege. *Theory, Culture & Society*, **17**(3): 26–54.

Marcus, G.E. (1994) What comes (just) after 'Post'?: the case of ethnography. In *Handbook of Qualitative Research* (Denzin, N.K. & Lincoln, Y.S., eds). Sage Publications, Thousand Oaks, CA.

May, T. (1999) Reflexivity and sociological practice. *Sociological Research Online*, **4**(3), http://www.socresonline.org.uk/socresonline/4/3/may.html

May, T. (2000) Reflexivity in social life and sociological practice: a rejoinder to Roger Slack. *Sociological Research Online*, **5**(1), http://www.socresonline.org.uk/5/1/may.html

Murphy, P.D. (2002) The anthropologist's son (or, living and learning in the field). *Qualitative Inquiry*, **8**(2), 246–62.

Paget, M.A. (1995) Performing the text. In *Representation in Ethnography* (Van Maanen, J., ed.). Sage Publications, Thousand Oaks, CA.

Parker, I. (1992) *Discourse Dynamics: Critical Analysis for Social and Individual Psychology.* Routledge, London.

Pels, D. (2000) Reflexivity: One step up. *Theory, Culture & Society*, **17**(3), 1–25.

Pollock, D. (1998) Performing writing. In *The Ends of Performance* (Phelan, P. & Lane, J., eds). New York University Press, New York.

Potter, J. (1996) *Representing Reality: Discourse, Rhetoric and Social Construction.* Sage Publications, London.

Potter, J. & Wetherell, M. (1987) *Discourse & Social Psychology: Beyond Attitudes and Behaviour.* Sage Publications, London.

Reason, P. (1988) (ed.) *Human Inquiry in Action.* Sage Publications, London.

Rheinharz, S. (1992) *Feminist Methods in Social Research.* Oxford University Press, New York.

Richardson, L. (1994) Writing: a method of inquiry. In *Handbook of Qualitative Research* (Denzin, N. & Lincoln, Y., eds). Sage Publications, Thousand Oaks, CA.

Rosaldo, R. (1993, first published 1989) Introduction: grief and a headhunter's rage. In

Culture and Truth: The Remaking of Social Analysis (Rosaldo, R., ed.). Routledge, London.

Seale, C. (1999) *The Quality of Qualitative Research*. Sage Publications, London..

Silverman, D. (1987) *Communication and Medical Practice*. Sage Publications, London.

Slack, R. (2000) Reflexivity or sociological practice: a reply to May. *Sociological Research Online*, 5(1), http://www.socresonline.org.uk/socresonline/5/1/slack.html

Smith, D.E. (1978) K is mentally ill: the anatomy of a factual account. *Sociology*, **12**, 23–53.

Stainton-Rogers, R., Stenner, P., Gleeson, K. & Stainton-Rogers, W. (1995) *Social Psychology: A Critical Agenda*. Polity Press, Cambridge.

Stanley, L. & Wise, S. (1993) *Breaking Out Again: Feminist Ontology and Epistemology*, 2nd edn. Routledge, London.

Taylor, C. & White, S. (2000) *Practising Reflexivity in Health and Welfare*. Open University Press, Buckingham.

Tyler, S.A. (1987) *The Unspeakable: Discourse, Dialogue, and Rhetoric in the Postmodern World*. University of Wisconsin Press, Madison.

Wetherell, M. & Maybin, J. (1996) The distributed self: a social constructionist perspective. In *Understanding The Self* (Stevens, R., ed.). Sage/Open University Press, London.

White, S. (1997) Beyond retroduction? Hermeneutics, reflexivity and social work practice. *British Journal of Social Work*, **27**(6), 739–53.

Wilkinson, S. (1988). The role of reflexivity in feminist psychology. *Women's Studies International Forum*, **11**, 493–502.

Woolgar, S. (1980) Discovery: logic and sequence in scientific text. In *The Social Process of Scientific Investigation*. (Knorr, K., Krohn, R. & Whitely, R., eds). Reidel, Dordrecht, Netherlands.

PART II

Personal Reflexivity

Most versions of reflexivity involve an examination of researcher preconceptions and motivations pertaining to the research question(s). One can quite easily acknowledge 'academic' reasons for pursuing a particular line of enquiry (gaps in the literature etc.), but taking time to scrutinise subjective investment in the research topic, including how the research question is initially formulated, can yield valuable, sometimes surprising, fruit. For example, a decision to study gender stereotyping in television advertisements for children's toys might well be (partially) prompted by the researcher's recollections and emotions pertaining to childhood experiences (perhaps s/he was only permitted to play with 'gender-appropriate' toys?) or current experience of parenthood (perhaps surprised and disappointed by her/his child's toy preferences?). Once such insights into such personal interests are identified, this can help with clarifying the research focus (on specific products, target age groups etc.). Including personal motivations as well as academic rationales in research reports can thus contextualise the research further and even refine research questions.

But we want to move beyond definitions of personal reflexivity as mere reflection on subjective thoughts and feelings experienced during the research process. Personal reflexivity also encompasses situating the researcher and his/her knowledge-making practices within relevant contexts, whether interpersonal, institutional or cultural. Thus, some chapters here connect researcher subjectivity to the interpersonal field and demonstrate how our experiences as researchers are affected by our encounters with research participants. Other chapters locate the researcher within wider disciplinary and societal contexts, thus suggesting that research-related activities which appear to be dictated by personal agenda are, partially at least, shaped by other forces beyond the individual.

In Chapter 3, Maso concentrates on the construction of the research question and argues that researchers should ask 'true' questions. By this he means questions which are personally relevant, which provoke 'passion' and which, therefore, initiate a meaningful research endeavour. Researchers are thus encouraged to invest effort in producing appropriate research questions, and Maso offers several fascinating examples, some from the history and philosophy of science, concerning the importance of passionate enquiry. Next, in Chapter 4, McKay, Ryan and Sumsion argue for the benefits of a research stance which involves personal reflection. This intriguing contribution offers three distinct narratives which depict how reflexivity became a possibility, then a reality, for these three qualitative researchers, each with different levels of experience in the field. Becoming reflexive is shown to be a fraught process – and many researchers will relate to their struggles – but one which entails personal and professional satisfaction. A co-written final section, compiled through dialogue, then develops a shared perspective on reflexivity.

In contrast, Ballinger in Chapter 5 considers researcher subjectivity in relation to the researcher selecting, or being assigned, different identities and responsibilities between research contexts. Drawing upon her research on older people and 'falling', she reflects on her treatment by health care professionals, health service users and academic colleagues while performing research-related activities. Her reflections are creatively presented via a present-tense 'reflexive voice' which uses discourse analytic concepts to help unpack the significance of these relative positionings.

Chapter 6 by Harper also considers discourse analytic work, with the focus this time on the researcher's knowledge-making practices. Reflecting on his study of 'paranoia', he examines researcher subjectivity as defined (and constrained) within historical, cultural and medical texts about paranoia and suspicion. Various assumptions and practices linked to discourse analysis are made available and discussed with reference to the author's experience in a form of methodological reflexivity. One of the strengths of this chapter is in opening up the process of doing discourse analysis to critical scrutiny – something rarely attempted in the literature.

Personal reflection, however, is often prompted by encounters with other people, including research participants. In Chapter 7, Doane powerfully advocates a form of reflexivity which is relational and beyond the personal. Her focus is on the experience of pain – on the part of both research participants and researchers. Instead of dealing with other people's pain by professional detachment or avoidance, researchers are invited to 'stay with' the pain and 'be' present, thereby experiencing a more rewarding engagement. The researcher's own experience of pain can also be enabled by this research orientation, and, in turn, the research process may be enriched.

CHAPTER 3

Necessary subjectivity: exploiting researchers' motives, passions and prejudices in pursuit of answering 'true' questions

Ilja Maso

Positioning the self: author's story

Earlier in my life, my research interests focused on ethnomethodology; I conducted doctoral research in that area and published a number of papers. At first, I found it novel and interesting to investigate the constructed character of our everyday and scientific rationality. But after a while I became aware of the limitations of ethnomethodology – it became a sterile enterprise for me. While investigating 'the existing', ethnomethodology seemed to refrain from developing new ideas and possibilities. I decided to quit the field and became involved in a different mode of qualitative research – a mode which concentrated on 'boundary subjects' such as coincidence, spirituality and paranormality. However, ethnomethodology has left deep marks in my thinking. For instance, I am still convinced that facts, reality, truth, objectivity, validity, reliability and consistency are constituted by the ordering practices of scientists, and that every rule has an 'etcetera clause', i.e. that every rule is incomplete insofar as it is formulated apart from the situation in which it has been or will be applied. The root of my idea of *necessary subjectivity* as a complement to both 'the rules of a method' and to 'validity and reliability' can probably be traced back to this conviction.

For me, reflexivity has always been the ethnomethodological maxim that the rationality of an event is constituted by the rationality of the practices that constitute that event and vice versa. It was a discovery for me that the reflexivity used in this book is not far removed from the ethnomethodological notion. There is, however, one big difference. Not everybody claims that these practices are or have been rational. I do.

In my role as Professor of the Theory of Science at the University for Humanistics in Utrecht, The Netherlands, I maintain a special interest in the boundaries of science and rationality (or normality). Specifically, I maintain scientific practices today are, in fact, disguised *social practices*. All too often science – the growth of knowledge – is directed at the preservation of the institutional and power structures of its own scientific community.

Introduction

Subjectivity is an inevitable part of the research process. Every experienced researcher knows that the rules of a method can never be applied to every question in every situation. Rules have to be interpreted, time and time again, to discover how they can be applied in a particular situation to answer a specific question. For instance, Garfinkel has shown that for professional sociological researchers, 'their concerns are for what is decidable "for practical purposes", "in light of this situation", "given the nature of actual circumstances", and the like', (Garfinkel, 1967, p.7; see also Lynch *et al.*, 1983).

In many cases this interpretation is not enough. Method, question and situation often have to be supplemented or changed totally, or partly ignored, or replaced by other approaches, questions or situations. None of this is exclusively executed by reason. Researchers bring with them their own emotions, intuitions, experiences, meanings, values, commitments, presuppositions, prejudices and personal agendas, their position as researchers and their spontaneous or unconscious reactions to subjects and events in the field. The discrepancies between the ethnographic studies of Samoan society by Mead (1928) and Freeman (1983) and those between Redfield (1930) and Lewis (1951) on the Mexican village Tepotzlán, for instance, are imputed to differences in perspective and temperament between the different researchers (Papousek, 1981, p.27; Kloos, 1983). It is no exaggeration to maintain that research is, to a large extent, a subjective enterprise kept reasonably in check by a number of more or less general methodological rules and considerations.

Because these predominantly subjective contributions may lead to systematic and random errors, they are generally considered to be harmful to the validity and reliability of research. True, sometimes qualitative research can seem to be more lenient to the demands of validity and reliability than in quantitative research. But even here, validity and reliability often remain important regulative principles. Guba and Lincoln's (1989) criteria of credibility, transferability and dependability, for instance, still refer to the conventions of internal and external validity, and reliability. They argue that these conventions are important because: '[t]he inquirer's [subjective] construction cannot be given privilege over that of anyone else' (1989, p. 238). In other words, qualitative researchers still 'do not advocate subjectively shaped products that need only meet the personal standards of their maker' (Jansen & Peshkin, 1992, p.716) or products that are the result of their personal whims and aberrations.

While subjectivity has acquired something of a bad name because of the 'scientific' demands of validity and reliability, researchers realise that the practice of research makes an element of subjectivity inescapable. This is why inquirers, through the use of reflexivity, are required to 'come clean' about how subjective and intersubjective elements have impinged on the research process in order to increase the integrity and trustworthiness of their research (Finlay, 2002). In this chapter, I argue that reflexivity is not only a way to 'come clean' about the influence of subjectivity on qualitative research, but that it can also function as an instrument to improve the quality of the research. In order to explore this dual role of subjectivity, the early stages of qualitative research are discussed with reference to the formulation of the research question, the generation of a theoretical framework and the mode of approach of the research subject.

The formulation of the research question

The importance of the research question cannot be overestimated. It is not enough to simply pose a question. As Peirce argues:

> 'Some philosophers have imagined that to start an inquiry it was only necessary to utter a question . . . and have even recommended us to begin our studies with questioning everything! But the mere putting of a proposition into the interrogative form does not stimulate the mind to any struggle after belief. There must be a real and living doubt, and without this all discussion is idle' (Peirce, 1955, p.11).

In order that research really involves the search for something, the question must be 'true', i.e. it must be the expression of a real and living doubt (see also Maslow, 1969, p.134). This means, firstly, that it is a question the researchers are eager to know the answer to. If the question originates from somebody else (e.g. a client), researchers should work out for themselves if they are able to appropriate this question, i.e. if they see it as an expression of what is a real and living doubt *to them*. Only then will they acquire the passion, the emotional investment, that 'provides the motivating force for the endless hours of intense, often gruelling, labor' (Keller, 1998, p.198; see also Maslow, 1969, p.110).[1] To be a true question means, secondly, that the answer to what is in question is not settled (Gadamer, 1988, p.326), i.e. that there exists no scientific literature that already answers the question convincingly.

As the expression of a real and living doubt, a 'true' question points to both limitation and openness: 'It implies the explicit establishing of presuppositions, in terms of which can be seen what still remains open' (Gadamer, 1988, p.327). These presuppositions do not indicate preliminary answers, but represent the

---

[1] This does not alter the fact that the French sociologist Pierre Bourdieu could be right in asserting that researchers 'consider as important and interesting that which stands a good chance of being recognized by others as important and interesting', i.e. that researchers engage themselves in certain questions 'in conscious or unconscious anticipation of their average chance of yielding a profit' (Bourdieu, 1989, p. 182).

situation in which the question has been asked, i.e. the motives, beliefs and conceptual framework from which the question has originated (Gadamer, 1986a, b). It is this situation which represents the sense of the question, the direction 'in which alone the answer can be given if it is to be meaningful' (Gadamer, 1988, p. 326). In other words, motives, beliefs and the conceptual framework open up the range of possible answers and thus the direction in which to look for them. In order to know what could be relevant, to overcome 'the fluid indeterminacy of the direction in which it is pointing' (Gadamer, 1988, p.327), every researcher has to know what motivated the research question, which beliefs are behind it and of which conceptual framework it is an expression. To this end, researchers must interrogate themselves and/or their clients.

A good way to do this is to use the 'why-interview' (Maso, 1984; Stuyling de Lange & Maas-de Waal, 1986). The first question in this interview seeks to reveal the various concepts that the question contains. The second asks why it is important for the researchers to ask this particular question. The answer here leads to further elucidation of the concepts the question contains (if necessary) and of the importance of the question to the researchers. This process is continued until it is completely clear what concepts the researchers are using, why the earlier formulated question is so important to them *and* whether the formulated question is a proper 'translation' of what is important to the researchers (see Maso & Smaling, 1998).

By way of example, I take the question a student started with when he wanted to do a qualitative research project. His question was: 'How do professional drivers manage to stay calm in traffic?' I then asked him what he meant by the following concepts: 'a professional driver', 'to manage to stay calm' and 'traffic'. On the basis of his answers, I *reformulated* his research question and verified with him that this was the 'correct' question. We then had the following discussion (which I have constructed retrospectively):

Interviewer: Why is this question so important to you?
Student: I think when I get insight into it, it will be possible to train other drivers to stay more calm in traffic.
I: Yes, I see the importance of that, but I would like to know why the question is so important to *you*. What has it to do with *you*?
S: You mean if I, personally, want to know how to stay calm in traffic?
I: Something like that.
S: What do you mean? Are there other possibilities that could have something to do with me?
I: I don't know. The only thing I would like to know is what the question has to do with you.
S: [after a rather long silence] Well, yes, from time to time I am a bit aggressive in traffic and that is something I blame myself for. I try not to, but it seems that I cannot drive without becoming aggressive.

I: So, it is important to you to avoid becoming aggressive in traffic?

S: Yes, because I realise that I am angry about things people do – things that I've often done myself or still do. But also, because, from time to time, I do something dangerous when I'm angry.

I: Could you give me an example?

S: Well, from time to time, there is this motorbike that drives in the middle of the road, making it impossible for cars to overtake it. At least, as long as there are oncoming cars. When at last I succeed in passing this bloke, I'm sometimes so worked up that I try to force him to the side of the road where he belongs. In retrospect, I realise that I could have caused him to collide with me or with someone else. And suppose that, because of that, he becomes an invalid or worse. I'm sure I would blame myself for it for the rest of my life. And all that because of something of no real importance.

I: Whereas you, sometimes, have also driven in the middle of the road, making it impossible for cars to pass you?

S: Well, yes, I've never had a motorbike but in the past I've cycled two or three abreast, making it impossible for a car to overtake us.

I: OK. If I understand you, you don't want to become aggressive, certainly not to the extent of being a danger to others and perhaps to yourself?

S: Yes, that is very important to me.

I: But, as far as I can see it, this doesn't figure in your research question. If the result of your research were to be that only those professional drivers stay in business who are calm by nature, you wouldn't have got an answer to what seems to be your real question.

S: Yes, you're right. It would be better to ask how car drivers can avoid becoming so aggressive that they become a danger to other road-users.

I: Yes, something like that.

S: One way could be that they learn to be less aggressive or not aggressive at all.

I: Yes, certainly.

Reading this, I can imagine that I seem to be detached, remote and authoritarian, and that this way of questioning looks like the way endlessly inquisitive children are sometimes pestering their parents. This is both the result of the fact that the text is a reconstruction of an actual dialogue, and of the fact that the attitude in which I do this interview is omitted in the text. In this kind of enterprise my general attitude is that of someone who, hesitating, uncertain but highly interested, is trying to find his way to the underlying motive. This makes it possible to use the why-interview with clients and even in everyday life situations, as my experience and those of others have shown. By using the why-interview, it became clear what this student meant by : 'a professional driver', 'to manage to stay calm', 'traffic' and 'aggressiveness'. In his answer, he revealed the beliefs underlying his question: that you can train drivers to stay calm, that he cannot drive without becoming aggressive, that he does dangerous things to other road users when he is aggressive, etc. He also uncovered what was, for him, his 'true' question.

However, it is not enough that a question is true from the point of view of the researcher – it has also to be true in the eyes of the scientific community. As we have already seen, this involves establishing that the answer to what is in question has not been settled already. This is done by studying the relevant scientific literature, and, if that seems to be insufficient, the non-scientific literature and/or by consulting people likely to have the relevant knowledge and experience. The outcome will be either that the research question has already been answered or that the question is a true question, i.e. that there exists genuine doubt as to what the possible answer could be. In the case of the latter, three important things will have happened to most researchers during the course of the process. Firstly, irrespective of whether the research question originated from themselves or from somebody else, they will have developed a keener, even passionate, interest in a possible answer to their question and, consequently, in the subject of their research. In other words, the question will have become even more true to them. Secondly, they will have been confronted by different preliminary answers, half-answers or leads to answers that, as will be shown, can be used as elements of the theoretical framework that will be constructed. Thirdly, they will have been confronted by some or most of their own ideas, assumptions, presuppositions and prejudices. In short, they will have discovered their own attitude to their proposed topic. Some historical examples help to emphasise the point.

Passion: an intermezzo

Two pertinent examples from the history of science come from Descartes and Goodyear.

René Descartes

Already during his education at the Royal Jesuit College of La Flèche, Descartes had discovered about philosophy that 'there is not a single thing of which it treats which is not still in dispute, and nothing, therefore, which is free from doubt' (Descartes, 1958, p.98). He considered, 'how many diverse opinions regarding one and the same matter are upheld by learned men, and that only one of all these opinions can be true' (1958, p.98). As regards the other sciences, inasmuch as they borrow their principles from philosophy, he judged that 'nothing solid can have been built on foundations so unstable' (1958, p.98). It was due to these disappointments that Descartes (as he put it) became 'obsessed by the eager desire to learn to distinguish the true from the false' (1958, p.99). In other words, Descartes acquired a true question and, with that, the passion to look for an answer that would convince him. 'For this reason', he writes, 'as soon as my age allowed of my passing from under the control of my teachers, ... I spent the remainder of my youth in travel, visiting courts and armies, in intercourse with men of diverse dispositions and callings.' In his search for answers to his question however, he found, 'almost as much diversity ... [as he] had previously found in the opinions of the philosophers' (1958, p.99). That is why he resolved to withdraw as far as possible from his country and his books to be able to take himself as the subject of study, and to employ all the powers of his mind in choosing the path that would lead him to true knowledge. The rest is history. After a search of five years and with the help of a visionary dream, he succeeded in developing a method which, after he had tested it for nine years, enabled him to slowly but surely progress with the search for 'truth' (1958, p. 95).

Charles Goodyear

After discovering rubber in the early sixteenth century, the Europeans found no important use for it, 'because it became soft and sticky at higher temperatures and stiff and brittle at lower temperatures' (Roberts, 1989, p.53). The young Charles Goodyear:

> 'became fascinated by the possibility of making rubber impervious to temperature changes so that it would be useful in many ways. This fascination became a compulsion that devoured Goodyear's health and the little wealth that he and his family had between 1830–39. During this period Goodyear was in debtor's prison more than once; he became dependent on relatives for food and shelter, but still his obsession persisted. ... After many unsuccessful and unscientific attempts to treat rubber, one of which involved mixing it with sulphur, he accidentally allowed a mixture of rubber and sulphur to touch a hot stove. To his surprise, the rubber did not melt but only charred slightly, as a piece of leather would' (Roberts, 1989, p.54).

This was the turning point that led to the discovery of the process of vulcanisation to make rubber impervious to temperature changes.

Both examples show that in many cases the answer to a question can only be found by an intensive and often sustained search. If that search is not supported by a passionate wish to acquire an answer that is satisfying to the questioner (and to the scientific community), it is very hard and sometimes impossible to keep going on. Neither Descartes nor Goodyear would have had the stamina to proceed if their question were not a 'true' one. Also, Newton was only able to accomplish what he set out to do because he had to have answers to his questions. The intensity and passion which fuelled his research led his laboratory assistant to remark: 'What his aim might be, I was not able to penetrate into, but his pains, his diligence at these times, made me think he aimed at something beyond the reach of human art and industry' (Westfall, 1993, p. 141).

This stamina to go on does not exhaust the function of a true question and its accompanying passion. According to Polanyi, this passion also has a heuristic function:

'The heuristic impulse links our appreciation of scientific value [of the question] to a vision of reality, which serves as a guide to enquiry. Heuristic passion is also the mainspring of originality – the force that impels us to abandon an accepted framework of interpretation and commit ourselves, by the crossing of a logical gap, to the use of a new framework. Finally, heuristic passion will often turn (and have to turn) into *persuasive* passion, the mainspring of all fundamental controversy' (Polanyi, 1973, p.159).

The examples of Descartes and Goodyear exemplify the heuristic function of their passion. Both saw reality as hiding a truth that exists by itself and that can therefore be discovered. Both used unconventional means to accomplish this fate and both, after having found what they were looking for, were convinced that they really had found the truth, and they acted accordingly. In other words, it was their subjectivity, in the face of reality, method and truth, that helped them make their discoveries. This subjectivity, according to Polanyi, is necessary because:

'A result obtained by applying strict rules mechanically, without committing anyone personally, can mean nothing to anybody. Desisting henceforth from the vain pursuit of a formalized scientific method, commitment accepts in its place the person of the scientist as the agent responsible for conducting and accrediting scientific discoveries. The scientist's procedure is of course methodical. But his methods are but the maxims of an art which he applies in his own original way to the problem of his own choice' (1973, p. 311).[2]

This insight gives even more substance to the view stated at the beginning of this chapter, that *subjectivity is an inevitable part of the research process.*

Generating a theoretical framework

As researchers study the relevant scientific and, where necessary, non-scientific literature, and consult people who have the relevant knowledge and experience, they will encounter different preliminary answers, half-answers or leads to answers as well as their own ideas, assumptions, presuppositions and prejudices. These confrontations are important to the progress of qualitative research inasmuch as they are used as the building blocks of a theoretical framework. This will consist of hypotheses, assumptions and presuppositions (including prejudices). A theoretical framework is therefore a hotchpotch of knowledge, experiences, ideas etc., that are relevant to answering the research question. For instance, one of my

---

[2] See also Maslow, 1969, pp. 134–35.

students who wanted to discover what psychological factors make it difficult to reach decisions, constructed a theoretical framework including such 'hypotheses' as the following:

- Within a person there is a relation between doubting on the one hand and responsibility, control, stress and/or insecurity on the other.
- A person who has difficulty in making decisions is someone who asks too much of herself.
- The more important the consequences of a decision, the more difficult it is to take such a decision.

My student found the first hypothesis in the scientific literature; the second was one of her own ideas; and the third one came from the literature but reflected also one of her, until then, hidden ideas.

Beyond bringing together everything of relevance to the research question, a theoretical framework is important to formulate a topic list that gives direction to the collection of information ('data'). In the above example of investigating decision making, the researcher explored responsibility, control, stress, insecurity, asking too much of oneself, and the importance of the consequences of a decision throughout her collection of data.

A theoretical framework is also important because it directs the analysis. Roughly, the analysis consists of confronting a theoretical framework with the collected information. The first confrontation with the initial data set can result in the confirmation, negation, or change of the hypotheses, assumptions and/or presuppositions of the theoretical framework. It can also lead to the generation of new hypotheses etc., and even to a modified research focus. Subsequently, new information will be collected in situations, or from participants, that represent a reasonable chance that the information to be collected will supplement, confirm or rather falsify the changed theoretical framework. This information, again, could lead to changes of the theoretical framework, and so on. In principle, this process will be continued until the theoretical framework no longer needs to be changed because no new information could be dragged up that makes a further change necessary (Maso & Smaling, 1998, pp.117–22). This stage is known as 'saturation' in the grounded theory literature (Glaser & Strauss, 1967).

In the case of the investigation of decision making, the idea that 'someone who has difficulty making decisions is someone who asks too much of herself' had to be withdrawn after the second interview. The researcher acknowledged this:

'After the first interview this item seemed still tenable. Looking into the second interview I found out what I really meant by "asking too much of yourself". It refers to two things, that is, "to want everything" and "to want everything your own way". Because I could subsume these meanings under two other hypotheses this item as such was abandoned.'

To sum up, it may be said that this kind of theoretical framework in qualitative research has many advantages: it brings together everything of relevance to the research question; it gives direction to the empirical collection of information via the (changing) topic list; it makes analysis more easy and enjoyable than tiresome conceptual work that is implied by the methods recommended in Spradley (1979), Strauss and Corbin (1990) and Miles and Huberman (1984, 1994); and it shows the contribution of the research in question to existing theoretical and practical notions because of the difference between the original framework and that developed at the end of the research. However, the most important advantage is the outcome of the 'forced' reflexivity caused by the confrontation with literature and experts and the exposure of the more or less hidden ideas, assumptions, presuppositions and prejudices of the researchers. By making these procedures part of the theoretical framework, researchers are able not only to 'test' their subjective beliefs but also to avoid the danger of being blind to information not compatible with their cherished theories (Maso & Smaling, 1998). The existence of these theories will, of course, be reflected by the theoretical framework – the subjective beliefs of the researchers could then constitute a necessary counterbalance to these theories and a key to new insights. In the example of the investigation of decision making, the idea that a person who has 'difficulty in making decisions is someone who asks too much of herself' was withdrawn. However, by subsuming it under another hypothesis, a new insight was generated: that someone who has problems with making a decision is someone who wants to exclude nothing, i.e. that he or she is someone who wants to keep all options open.

Staying open and aware

As we have seen, a 'true' question implies, on the one hand, the explicit establishing of presuppositions – the motives, beliefs and conceptual framework from which the question has originated – and on the other hand, the range of possible answers and thus the direction in which to look for them. A true question thus points to both limitation and openness. Both the limitation and the openness of a true question must be reflected in the attitude of the researchers. The limitations researchers impose on themselves should be flexible: no information should be excluded as long as there is a chance that it could be relevant to their search. As for openness, this means that they must be receptive to everything they encounter. This implies that:

> 'not only "the empirical reality" but all the preceding, accompanying and resulting thoughts, feelings, inspirations, intuitions, fantasies, images, etc. must be scrutinized. After all, the subjectivity of the researcher reflects the outcome of the meeting of his or her perspective on the research situation

and what that situation reveals within and because of this perspective' (Maso, 1995, p.17).

An important part of what researchers find will not come from planned experiences or events. Whether because of selective perception (e.g. Postman and Bruner), the workings of the unconscious (e.g. Beth), the synchronicity between an inner experience and outer events (e.g. Jung), or the Idea of the Good (e.g. Plato), people who are passionately driven by a real question often encounter accidental events, corporal changes and flashes of inspiration that can aid them in finding answers. The history of science and technology is replete with examples of these kind of occurrences (see, for instance, Maso, 1997). In terms of reflexivity, this means that researchers must train themselves to become aware of everything that could constitute a contribution to their search for answers to their question. They must not only be aware, but also act accordingly. Depending on the nature of the occurrence, this action can extend from writing an idea down for subsequent use, to following it up. During the regular sessions in which students exchange information about the progress they are making with their research, they report frequently that they have found by accident a book, a respondent, a research situation or information that is useful in that stage of their research. Their concern to answer their true question makes them generally aware of opportunities that could further the search for a satisfying answer.

Summary

By being reflexive about their own subjectivity, qualitative researchers can improve the quality of their research. If they make sure that their research question is the expression of a real and living doubt – by studying their own motives and the scientific literature – their search will be supported by a passionate wish to acquire answers satisfying both to them and to the scientific community. This passion can serve as a guide to enquiry; it can also lead to originality. It fuels a determination to become aware of everything that could contribute to the search for answers and it promotes persistence in the face of seemingly insurmountable problems. However, passion alone can potentially lead researchers into the wilderness. To avoid this, they have to know what motivated their research question, which beliefs are behind it and of which conceptual framework it is an expression. These motives and beliefs and this conceptual framework open up the range of possible answers to the research question and thus the direction in which to look for them.

This direction will also be indicated by a theoretical framework that consists of the different preliminary answers, half-answers or leads to answers that are found in the literature and of the ideas, assumptions, presuppositions and prejudices of the researchers that are (partly) the outcome of the forced reflexivity caused by their confrontation with the literature. By making these subjective beliefs part of the theoretical framework, researchers are able not only to know which way they want to go, but also to 'test' these beliefs and, in this way, to avoid the danger of being blind to information not compatible with their cherished theories that are also part of the theoretical framework. Their subjective beliefs can constitute a necessary counterbalance to these theories and a key to new insights.

References

Bourdieu, P. (1989) Het wetenschappelijk veld. (1976) In *Opstellen Over Smaak, Habitus en het Veldbegrip* (Bourdieu, P., ed.). Van Gennep, Amsterdam.

Descartes, R. (1958) Discourse on method: of rightly conducting the reason and of seeking for truth in the sciences (1637) In *Philosophical Writings* (Descartes, R., ed.). The Modern Library, New York.

Finlay, L. (2002) 'Outing' the researcher: the provenance, process and practice of reflexivity. *Qualitative Health Research*, 12(4), 531–45.

Freeman, D. (1983) *Margaret Mead and Samoa*. Harvard University Press, Cambridge, MA.

Gadamer, H.-G. (1986a) Was ist Wahrheit? (1957) In *Gesammelte Werke. Band 2. Hermeneutik II: Wahrheit und Methode* (Gadamer, H.-G., ed.). J.C.B. Mohr (Paul Siebeck), Tübingen.

Gadamer, H.-G. (1986b) Begriffsgeschichte als Philosophie. (1970) In *Gesammelte Werke. Band 2. Hermeneutik II: Wahrheit und Methode* (Gadamer, H.-G., ed.). J.C.B. Mohr (Paul Siebeck), Tübingen.

Gadamer, H.-G. (1986c) Mensch und Sprache. (1966) In *Gesammelte Werke. Band 2. Hermeneutik II: Wahrheit und Methode* (Gadamer, H.-G., ed.). J.C.B. Mohr (Paul Siebeck), Tübingen.

Gadamer, H.-G. (1988) *Truth and Method* (1960). Sheed and Ward, London.

Garfinkel, H. (1967) *Studies in Ethnomethodology*. Prentice-Hall, Englewood Cliffs, NJ.

Glaser, B.G. & Strauss, A. (1967) *The Discovery of Grounded Theory: Strategies for Qualitative Research*. Aldine de Gruyter, Hawthorne, NY.

Guba, E.G. & Lincoln, Y.S. (1989) *Fourth Generation Evaluation*. Sage Publications, London.

Jansen, G. & Peshkin, A. (1992) Subjectivity in qualitative research. *The Handbook of Qualitative Research in Education*, 681–725 (LeCompte, M.D., Preissle Goetz, J. & Millroy, W.L., eds). Academic Press, London).

Keller, E.F. (1998) *A Feeling for the Organism: The Life and Work of Barbara McClintock* (1983). W.H. Freeman and Company, New York.

Kloos, P. (1983) De aanval op Margaret Mead. *Intermediair*, 19(28), 1–7.

Lewis, O. (1951) *Life in a Mexican Village*. University of Illinois Press, Illinois.

Lynch, M.E., Livingston, E. & Garfinkel, H. (1983) Temporal order in laboratory work. In *Science Observed: Perspectives on the Social Study of Science* (Knorr-Cetina, K.D. & Mulkay, M., eds). Sage Publications, London.

Maslow, A.H. (1969) *The Psychology of Science: A Reconnaissance* (1966). Henry Regnery Company, Chicago.

Maso, I. (1984) *Verklaren in het Dagelijks Leven: Een Inleiding in Etnomethodologisch Onderzoek*. Wolters-Noordhoff, Groningen.

Maso, I. (1995) Trifurcate openness. In *The Deliberate Dialogue: Qualitative Perspectives on the Interview* (Maso, I. & Wester, F., eds). VUBPress, Brussels.

Maso, I. (1997) *De Zin van het Toeval*. Ambo, Baarn.

Maso, I. & Smaling, A. (1998) *Kwalitatief Onderzoek: Praktijk en Theorie*. Boom, Amsterdam.

Mead, M. (1928) *Coming of Age in Samoa*. W. Morrow, New York.

Miles, M.B. & Huberman, M. (1984, 1994) *Qualitative Data-analysis: A Sourcebook of New Methods*. Sage Publications, London.

Papousek, D.A. (1981) Op het land waar het leven goed is. *Intermediair*, 17(27), 23–31, 39.

Peirce, C.S. (1955) The fixation of belief (1877). In *Philosophical Writings of Peirce* (1940) (Buchler, J., ed.). Dover Publications, New York.

Polanyi, M. (1973) *Personal Knowledge: Towards a Post-Critical Philosophy*. Routledge & Kegan Paul, London.

Redfield, R. (1930) *Tepotzlán, a Mexican Village*. University of Chicago Press, Chicago, Illinois.

Roberts, R.M. (1989) *Serendipity: Accidental Discoveries in Science*. John Wiley & Sons, New York.

Spradley, J.P. (1979) *The Ethnographic Interview*. Holt, Rinehart & Winston, New York.

Strauss, A.L. & Corbin, J. (1990) *Basics of Qualitative Research. Grounded Theory: Procedures and Tactics*. Sage Publications, New York.

Stuyling de Lange, J. & Maas-de Waal, C.J. (1986) De etnomethodologie en het hermeneutisch pragmatisme van Rorty: het abnormale karakter van Garfinkels conflictmethodologie. *Kennis en Methode*, **10**, 286–98.

Westfall, R.S. (1993) *The Life of Isaac Newton*. Cambridge University Press, Cambridge.

CHAPTER 4

Three journeys towards reflexivity

Elizabeth McKay, Susan Ryan and Thelma Sumsion

Positioning the selves: authors' stories

Each of us has a background in occupational therapy and we now work in universities, primarily in postgraduate programmes. The three of us are in the process of working towards completing our doctoral studies. This work reflects our different areas of interest and our diverse backgrounds. Thelma's research has defined the concept of client-centred practice from a UK perspective. Susan's area of study has built on her previous work on clinical reasoning development in practitioners. Elizabeth's thesis has centred on women and mental illness and therapists' perspectives of working with them. The following stories will help you see the journeys we have experienced so far in gaining our present stances on reflexivity.

Thelma was a novice qualitative researcher when she started her study. The methods used and the processes she encountered increased her awareness of the importance of reflecting on her role as researcher. From these experiences Thelma has learned some valuable lessons which she shares here. In contrast, Susan had worked with various qualitative methods over several years. It was only as her understanding of qualitative work deepened that she began to appreciate her influence on the research process as a whole, not only on the interpretive stages. Her section addresses the differences between reflection and reflexivity. Elizabeth's research was qualitative, using life history as a method (Atkinson, 1998). It focuses on the lived experience of women with enduring mental illness. Reflexivity was a core consideration from the outset as constructing and reconstructing another's life story was an interpretative act that required her to be aware of her presence in and on the research process.

For the purposes of this chapter we decided upon Mauthner and Doucet's (1998) definition of reflexivity as:

'. . . reflecting upon and understanding our own personal, political and intellectual autobiographies as researchers and making explicit where we are located in relation to our research respondents. Reflexivity also means acknowledging the critical role we play in creating, interpreting and theorizing data' (p. 121).

Introduction

You know how it is!... The three of us were at a conference on qualitative research methods, when one of us, Elizabeth to be precise, suggested collaborating on writing a chapter on reflexivity because we all had differing experiences and understandings of the construct.

As we put together the chapter we wished that we had been privy to its contents before we started our own research journeys instead of struggling in the dark on our own. On reflection, we realised that these personal roads of discovery were necessary and fruitful. In what follows, we map our personal research experiences and our deepening relationship with reflection and reflexivity.

We began by first asking how we each had developed our personal reflexive stance. We each realised that we had been using the concepts of reflection and reflexivity differently. Thelma as a relative novice needed to learn and be convinced about their use. Susan was experienced with reflection but needed to accommodate the notion of reflexivity. Elizabeth used both concepts at different levels. Maybe, as you read on, one or other of our stories will strike a chord with you.

Thelma's tentative steps towards reflexivity

When I started my research I was both sceptical and ignorant about reflexivity. My awareness and understanding grew, however, as my research progressed. I can now see three distinct stages in my growth. In the first, little reflection was involved. The objective of phase I of my study was to create the first draft of a definition of client-centred practice. It involved a Delphi study with occupational therapists from various regions of the United Kingdom. I had secured some funding for this phase which included the promise to complete this work within seven months. In hindsight, this was an unrealistic time frame. I was too busy completing tasks to think about what I was doing or my role in the research process. I knew I had only five years in which to complete a thesis on a part-time basis and my initial focus was on getting the job done.

In phase II, I conducted a series of groups with therapists from a variety of areas of practice in Greater London. I used the nominal group technique to prioritise components of client-centred practice and to gain the participants' views on the definition that had been created in phase I. As I transcribed the hours of audiotapes, I became increasingly aware of my role in these groups. I realised that my views sometimes dominated the participants' discussions (see Box 4.1).

During this second phase I also began to make field notes about the members in each group, the progress of the session and my opinions about the group and my performance in it (Pope & Mays, 2000). Gradually, I learned to make these notes

Box 4.1   Rethinking long-held beliefs

I had worked in client-centred practice for many years in Canada and had been at the forefront in developing this concept in practice. Therefore, I came to these groups with much experience and some ideas about the importance of this approach. In the groups, I was confused as the participants seemed to separate some key concepts that I believed went together. Overall, the therapists were in favour of the concept of partnership including the therapist and client working together in collaboration. However, they were less enthusiastic about including the concept of the client as an active participant within the team. Their position confused me, upset my equilibrium. Something I was so sure I understood, almost taking it for granted, was being challenged. It felt uncomfortable. This experience caused me to reconsider my stance and my long-held beliefs. As a result I had to change to accommodate my participants' perspectives.

Having strong convictions may have caused me to be defensive when my knowledge about client-centred practice was challenged by a group member who had completed a Master's level module on this topic. Significantly, I began to realise that my role as a researcher would have an impact on this study. As we were all occupational therapists, I reflected on my relationship with the participants and on what was really being said (Miles & Huberman, 1994). I also became aware of the subjectivity of myself as the researcher even though I was attempting to use a more objective structure (Frank, 1997). This is what Crabtree & Miller (1999) refer to as self-reflection. This involves being aware of yourself and how you are changed by the research process, as well as how you alter the process.

more reflective and less descriptive by including my thoughts and feelings rather than focusing on actions and events. For example, I initially began to record things that interrupted the sessions, such as alarm bells. Then, I progressed to reviewing group dynamics and my reactions to these. The participants' views of client-centred practice were often relatively narrow and I realised that I had to amend my perspective to include their understanding. I also learned to accept the confusion and uncertainty that was an integral part of reflection. At this time I also became aware of the importance of 'talking' to help me to reflect and become more reflexive. A new colleague, Elizabeth in fact, had joined our department and her willingness to listen to my ruminations and concerns about both my abilities and the depth of information I was obtaining, shed considerable light on my research process. For instance, up to this point, I had been bound by my research structure; now I was encouraged to think more freely about the people and their issues.

In phase III, I conducted open in-depth interviews with therapists and structured interviews with clients in an out-patient mental health setting to determine the opportunities for, and barriers to, implementing this definition. Transcribing the therapist interviews enhanced my ability to read and hear the data reflexively. Now I was able to see myself much more in the data and become aware of my role in generating it (Mason, 1996). For example, I was aware of some missed opportunities to obtain greater depth. I realised that I could not eliminate my role; rather I, as researcher, needed to monitor and discuss my influence on the research process and the interpretation of the data. Transcribing the tapes (as soon as possible after each session) also allowed me to reflect on my interactions with the participants as well as their perspectives – which frequently differed from mine (Carpenter, 2000). An example from my fieldnotes at the time recalls this questioning and its impact:

'Why, so far, are all the clients telling me things are great? Are they or am I just not asking the right questions to get at the true essence of client-centred practice? Or am I a stranger who might affect their access to the programme if they express concerns?'

I also became aware that my pace was slowing as I proceeded through this phase. Taking this extra time allowed me to contemplate and be open to new possibilities, for instance thinking in terms of metaphors (Pierson, 1998). One *metaphor* I developed was to conceptualise the place of the client in the treatment process in terms of the theatre, seeing the client as the leading actor and the other team members as the cast.

Now, in the midst of phase III, I am beginning to understand the importance of reflexivity in qualitative research while recognising that there is no definitive blueprint for its application (Mason, 1996). I am also moving towards an understanding of the importance of questioning my data and considering the distance between myself and my participants (Miles & Huberman, 1994; Pope & Mays, 2000).

I now understand the importance of my values and beliefs which underlie my approach to client-centred practice and how the credibility of my findings will rely on the resonance of this experience with all phases of the work (Wellington & Austin, 1996; Pope & Mays, 2000). I was initially unaware of the importance of reflection, finding it an elusive concept that I did not trust (Watson & Wilcox, 2000). There are still many steps to be taken before any level of mastery of the application of reflexivity has been reached. As I said in my notes:

'Initially, I didn't understand what reflexivity was. I am still not sure. But, I have learned the value of adopting a slower pace so there is time to consider different issues that arise and to do so from a variety of perspectives. Reflexivity is not concrete. In order to embrace it you have to give up tight control of your own process. This is not an easy thing to do without a large dose of confidence in yourself as a researcher.'

Three years later I am convinced of the value of reflection and reflexivity and am beginning to understand how important it is to allow *time and personal freedom* for this reflexivity to occur.

Susan's journey: interweaving reflection and reflexivity

Have you ever experienced hearing someone say something which you realise has made a profound impression on your thinking? This happened to me some years ago when I heard Della Fish speak about artistic practice. I had never heard that phrase before and neither had I heard of the model of reflection that she and her collaborators called 'Strands of Reflection' (Fish *et al.*, 1991). Reflection, she said, was the tool that helped practice be unique for the professional, distinct in its delivery and particular for the individual receiving therapy. Suddenly, I became aware that this work filled a gap in my understanding about practice. It was like finding a missing link or having a light bulb suddenly go on. This realisation led to a complete change of direction in my educational practice.

Briefly, Fish *et al.* (1991) recommend exploring a piece of practice using four different strands of reflection. The first strand tells the story and points out *critical incidents* of that narrative. The second strand causes the reflector to search for *generalised patterns* or ways of working that link with previous work so that you begin to see the way that you normally respond to circumstances. The third challenges the thinker to become aware of their *own values* and to imagine how these may have impacted on this piece of practice. The final strand looks to *the future* to see what should be altered if one was in a similar situation again.

This model delved into practice in a far deeper way than other models of reflection I had previously encountered. The metaphor of digging deeply around a topic appealed to me and became the catalyst that altered my thinking. I realised that this reflective method would give answers that went beyond the glib 'thinking about' ways of working that many people label as reflection. It became clear that it is necessary to revisit a specific piece of work, thinking about it from many perspectives in order to see it differently.

I understood that I, too, needed to be part of this way of working. It dawned upon me that reflection and reflexivity were distinct but intertwined. Originally, Fish told me that these strands should occur at the same time – the reflector needed to think about a piece of practice from different angles in order to gain different insights. Students, however, did not like this model when my colleagues and I tried to put it into practice. They found it tedious and did not achieve the intended depth of thinking. Slowly I realised that it was the *time element* that needed attention rather than the concept of the strands. An alternative approach might be to follow one strand through and not to attempt all four at the same time. If practice could be captured more naturally through writing, talking or recording at the end of each period then the first strand could be completed in a more natural way. Doing it like this did not allow for the critical incidents to be picked out but I could see with more time these could be done at the next stage. While more time-consuming, this process meant the reflector was engaging at a much deeper level. Obviously, reflecting like this must be used selectively for particular parts of practice. It is not realistic to work like this all the time. This method, therefore, lends itself to times when difficult or messy practice is being described or when deeper understanding is required. Interestingly, several years later Fish & Coles (1998) revised their own use of time with the strands. Time was needed in order to dwell on things.

These realisations have come slowly to me over a span of five years. During this period I have used different models of reflection for a variety of purposes (Schon, 1907, Boud & Walker, 1991), including in my research and teaching on clinical reasoning. I have thought a great deal about the use of reflection and have begun to develop some personal insight into reflexivity and its relationship with reflection.

Supervising postgraduate dissertations forced me to look again at the more personal meanings of reflexivity. Focusing on reflection was, in a sense, looking 'out there' even though the third strand had called for a look inward at personal values. I had always taken this to mean my values towards that piece of practice rather than seeing my roles and their effects on practice and on others. This insight came as a revelation to me. I was simultaneously aware that much thought and effort had helped me come to this point. As always, once you can 'see', it seems obvious. I then began to bring myself, my experiences and my thoughts into my work. I even began to write in such a way that I became part of the work as well. I experimented with these thinking and writing styles and published chapters and papers as a way of deepening my understanding. One of the most daring was a chapter where I used the Four Strands with a colleague. Telling the story about her early years we made links together with her present way of living and working (Denshire & Ryan, 2001). Although this was not my reflexivity but hers, it illustrated how we infuse our subjectivity into everything we do. I was now trying to make this explicit.

These new understandings formed the methodological base of my doctoral research (Ryan, 2003). Now realising that my own educational and life experiences had influenced my way of working, I wanted to find out how this applied to others' experiences. More specifically, I wanted to find out if life experiences were encouraged to flower during a professional training course. With this in mind I tracked the personal journeys of newly qualified occupational therapists from student to practitioner. By telling a story and then delving deeply into that narrative in successive layers *over a period of time*, the therapists would, I hoped, gain new insights: they might make links with their educational experiences, their life experiences and their ways of working. Further reflections on the original trigger point might prompt deeper awareness of themselves or of professional matters they might not otherwise have considered.

At this time the work of Foucault (1994) also intrigued me. He illustrated his work on medical perception with archaeological terms – again the metaphor of digging deeply and unearthing new discoveries. This was slightly different from reflectively dwelling on an aspect of work. I decided to combine the two in an attempt to elicit more discoveries and links. I wanted more critical self-awareness from those in the study and from myself. I wanted to see how my position (as a senior academic), my methods, and my roles as researcher, therapist and confidant impacted on my participants.

My participants came from two schools with different learning philosophies: one used traditional methods and the other problem-based learning (PBL). I was keen to see if these approaches had made any difference to the way they practised. Luckily, all fourteen who volunteered were experienced and of mature years; they brought a phenomenal richness of life with them.

My methodology had four layers. This meant that I met each participant four times over a period of five months. Their stories extended from their last placement to the first few months of working in their first setting. Interspersed with these four layers were other opportunities for myself and the participants to reflect on what was said. They were encouraged to reflect through a process of data collection that aimed to be an iterative and reiterative cycle. Work was sent out beforehand so that they could deliberate on what they would talk about. A tape recorder was left with each person for two weeks after the meetings in case they thought of other things they wished to add. Transcripts were returned to them so that they could pick out critical incidents and reflect on these further.

At the same time that my participants were reflecting on their interviews I, too, reflected – my own reflexivity was intertwined with theirs. Not wishing to influence the flow of their thoughts during the interviews, I mostly listened. I reflected on my own changing thought processes. The original conceptual frameworks that had been firmly settled in my mind now had to be cleared away to give me space to look afresh at what I was hearing. The therapists' stories became interlaced with my own.

Elizabeth's route to reflexivity: road maps don't help

I started my research recognising the importance of reflexivity to the research process. Drawing on past experiences I sought a research design which placed reflexivity at its core. Firstly, I valued methods that emphasised the search for personal understanding and meanings, for instance using a reflective journal. Secondly, I drew explicitly upon concepts such as reflective practice and clinical reasoning. Thirdly, I embraced opportunities for educational supervision and mentorship to enable personal and professional development (Hunter & Blair, 1999). My supervisors have continued to challenge my thinking and change my practice.

To locate myself in my research, first I utilised the model proposed by Boud and Walker (1991). They advocate that reflection, to enable effective learning, should occur before, during and after an event. The event, in this case, was the data collection phase of the study.

The *before* activities involved me identifying and focusing on my knowledge, skills and, importantly, my intent prior to the event. I was aware that my personal subjectivity would act as a lens for framing questions and viewing the resultant findings from a particular viewpoint. As an occupational therapist, I had worked with women with enduring mental illness in many contexts over several years. I have both theoretical and practical experience of the impact of mental illness on the lives of women. (I have, for example, witnessed how women have often been silenced by the mental health system by being labelled 'manipulative'.) It will come as no surprise that I sought to develop a method which placed the participants to the fore of the research where their stories could be heard and valued. The use of a grand tour question, 'tell me about your life history', in the first round of interviews, I hoped, would enable the women to share what they wished to share – in their own way, in their own voice, and without any other set questions from me driving the agenda.

The *during* activities place importance on the central task – in my case, the life history interview. During the interview situation there was a need for me to be aware of and notice what was occurring – specifically how was I interacting with the participants and influencing the process. To illuminate this I offer a reflection from my diary of one interview where Sarah revealed that she believed she had a multiple personality disorder – a diagnosis that has invoked much controversy in psychiatry. I was totally unprepared for this revelation:

'I became very aware of myself within the room, sitting on the floor near the recorder; I was monitoring my non-verbal communication, while simultaneously trying to hear what was being said and doing so in a way that was supportive and non-judgemental of her. Multiple personality disorder can lead to raised eyebrows in some arenas. Suddenly, I became aware of Sarah using "we", she had moved from "I" to "we" so naturally, so fluidly. I was surprised at this transition, but managed to ask her to expand on what she meant. She went on to explain further. I believe that if I had reacted differently, perhaps been more challenging or critical of her, she would have closed down this conversation and my understanding of her life would have remained unknown to me and a significant part of her life world would have been denied. Here my response to this important part of her life allowed further disclosure influencing the final outcome, the complexity and depth of her story. Being aware of my presence at that moment was vital.'

Finally, the *after* event, in this case post-interview, involved me recording my immediate feelings following the interview and then later returning to these and the transcripts to retrospectively examine the experience: giving consideration to what worked well, other ways of working and reviewing outcomes. For example, during the second round of interviews I made time to take each of the women through their life profile to ensure that they felt they had collaborated in the final product.

Beyond using this reflective model to explore what I personally and professionally brought to the study, I also sought to develop a collaborative relationship with my participants. The first step was to be open about my own background and interests. I was a woman researching other women's lives, a therapist and a qualitative researcher – all these identities intermingled. The struggle, at times, was to separate and identify the different influences on my study. Initially, the women were introduced to me as 'a researcher who was an occupational therapist'. Believing that these women might have had experiences of occupational therapy, I felt that my researcher persona should be to the fore – a different person entering their life story for very different reasons. At times during the interviews, I was aware of myself as an occupational therapist wishing to somehow make things better for the women. I cringed at some of their experiences at the hands of mental health professionals and was embarrassed that I, too, was part of this group. On a few occasions, I found myself empathising, sympathising and agreeing with the women. Their experiences were so vivid, so painful, that they demanded some kind of response – more than a knowing nod from a detached observer. For example, when Pat revealed that her sons had been sexually abused following her admission to hospital I felt the need to support her physically and shifted my position to be nearer to her. Being aware of such important moments and recording responses, I think, improves the credibility of the research.

Opie (1992) stresses the need for the researcher to recognise that her own processes impact on the research. As I began to read more feminist literature, I became aware that reflexivity in feminist research was taken for granted as an essential component. The need to recognise the 'power relationship' within research was openly acknowledged and steps were taken to empower participants within the process. I had considered reflexivity but not feminism, an omission that has since been addressed in my study.

To illustrate my current use of reflexivity further, I would like to share something of my experience of hearing Helen's story (see Box 4.2). (These reflections are constructed from notes recorded at the time as well as my present interpretation of her life.)

What I learned from this analytical process is that even though my research had methods for reflexivity built in, they would not necessarily work unless you *engaged with them*. The maps only offer routes towards reflexivity. Being reflexive involves me moving in and out of the data, revisiting and revising my own stance. It is a process that requires time, thinking space and, importantly, engagement. Helen taught me that there are many levels to reflexivity and that these need to be explored. While there is often an 'obvious' answer, it may be incorrect.

Box 4.2   Helen

Prior to the interview we had several telephone conversations. Helen was motivated to take part in the study and she wanted others to hear her story. I was eager to meet her. The first interview was unstructured as described above. Helen told her story. I heard a comprehensive narrative. Here was a woman who had experienced many difficulties in her life but nonetheless had worked hard, sometimes having three jobs simultaneously. She had fought for help for herself and others with mental health problems.

Nonetheless, I left the interview with a number of issues and a growing sense of discomfort. I recorded in my reflective journal that I had a nagging feeling that Helen's narrative seemed rehearsed: was this story what she had wanted me to hear? If so, what had she omitted and why? Importantly, it seemed to me, her husband and her only daughter rarely appeared in her story. In fact they seemed to play only 'bit parts' in her life. I wondered why?

As I transcribed the interview these issues remained unresolved. I worked on her transcript, firstly identifying the chronological events, and then, by using concept mapping, I began to conceptualise the major themes in Helen's life. But my initial impression of absence of her significant relationships was upheld. These 'gaps' formed questions for the follow-up interview: for example, her relationship with her daughter now and in the past, what life events had occurred, about her daughter's marriage, the grandchildren, more of her life with her husband. Meanwhile, Helen's verbatim transcript was returned to her for comment.

Sixteen months later, my second interview occurred. This was designed to have distinct components: a review of the chronological events, discussion of the concept map and questions relating to it and finally, retrospective questions and an opportunity for open discussion. However, it became apparent as soon as Helen came to her front door that things would not go according to my plan. She was a shadow of her former self. Since our last meeting Helen, 76 years old at the time of this interview, had undergone major surgery and was physically much weaker. Indeed, she was struggling to make her breakfast. I automatically put my researcher's role to one side as I helped her make her toast and tea. It seemed to me this was the least I could do, she seemed so weak and feeble. There was no way that as a caring human being, as a therapist, I could have watched her struggle when I was capable of assisting. I remember thinking, 'This isn't supposed to happen!'

With Helen settled, it became clear that she would retell her own story in her own way. My protocol quickly fell by the wayside. My anxiety rose about my incomplete data set and for a time I was unable to attend to Helen. However, as I began to tune into Helen's new story my anxiety slowly dispersed. She told a familiar story but with much more detail and depth than before. I would never have got that depth, I would never have got that narrative, if I had reasserted my own protocol over Helen's or if I had strictly maintained my researcher's role on my arrival. Perhaps my willingness to help her, be with her, changed the relationship.

Cont.

Box 4.2   *Cont.*

Helen now spoke of her guilt with regards to her husband and her daughter. She felt that she had never been a proper wife. She didn't like sex, so sex was rare and as a result she felt unable to take her husband's money, as she didn't 'deserve' it. So she had several jobs to enable her to have some measure of financial independence. Because her daughter became an alcoholic, Helen felt that somehow she failed to be a good mother and was perhaps responsible for her daughter's drinking problem. None of this had been raised previously . . . my gaps had been filled and my questions answered.

As I left, I felt that, for Helen, the research process and her general state of health had come together to create a moment where she could set the record straight, acknowledge it and move on. Her future was uncertain, but it seemed she was preparing for her death. This was uncomfortable for me to hear and painful for Helen to tell. But my understanding of her life was completely altered as a result of this encounter.

Discussion and sharing

These personal accounts have shown how each of us has experienced our complicated journey towards understanding and applying reflexivity. Thelma's account highlights the tentative steps she followed towards realising the importance of reflexivity to her role as a researcher. Susan's journey led her beyond a predetermined model to combine similar yet different constructs that unearthed richer data. Elizabeth's increasing awareness of reflexivity emphasises the importance of reflection-in-action.

Despite the differences in our journey, some commonalities have emerged:

- The individuality of application is evident – there are many routes that can be followed. Each journey reflects the individual's situatedness and biography.
- Each of us has highlighted the need for active engagement in thinking about, and through, our interactions throughout the research journey. Space and place are necessary for this to occur.
- Reflexivity is a dynamic experience that ebbs and flows.
- Reflexivity requires the researcher to be both immersed in the data and the research process, but also to be able to draw back and contemplate what is occurring.
- Involvement in the reflexive process results in changes in our thinking structures, perspectives, perceptions and in our views in relation to research.

Our discussions when bringing this chapter together also revealed a further commonality – the theme of *time* kept appearing in various guises. We seemed to be viewing it different ways: historical, developmental and spatial.

Historical time

We became aware that we had completed our professional education in different eras. Both Thelma and Susan had been schooled in the positivistic way of thinking that was characteristic of the late 1970s and early 1980s. Structure, logic and analysis guided their views of practice. These methods sat alongside the quantitative research paradigm that they were taught. In contrast, Elizabeth's undergraduate experience in the late 1980s and her postgraduate studies in the early 1990s encompassed qualitative research. Reflection was an integral part of these new methods that were being used increasingly by occupational therapy researchers in this era.

Developmental time

There is contemporary debate about where reflection should be introduced in undergraduate education. Atkinson & Claxton (2000) argue that learners need time to consolidate knowledge before they can reflect upon it. This is in marked contrast to previous thinking which suggested reflection should begin at the inception of a course. These debates notwithstanding, reflection and reflexivity do need to be developed and this, in our experience, happens over an extended period of time.

We began to appreciate that our understanding had altered quite dramatically over time. We all became aware that the construct of reflection had been our starting point in our development as educators and practitioners. Focusing on our practice we had used reflection through questioning, discussing, analysing and reviewing our work. Although our feelings and values were part of that process we had not grasped the subtleties between reflection and reflexivity. In particular, we understand the value of looking at ourselves in far greater detail, especially as it relates to our positions, the impact on and our efforts within the research process.

Spatial time

We realised that we required time and space, which we have called spatial time, to allow the process of reflexivity to happen. Time is an essential element in the 'here and now' but it also embraces both past events and future considerations. Reflexivity is not time limited and it has no endpoint. Becoming more reflexive requires the passage of time. It also needs to be nurtured in order to blossom.

Summary

In conclusion, this chapter has told of our three different journeys towards reflexivity. In sharing our narratives, we have reaffirmed our commitment to reflexivity as an essential element of the qualitative research process. We argue for reflexivity as a way to engage with people that allows the richness of their lives to be revealed. While the reflexive process can be rewarding it can also be frustrating. The confusion and muddle that occur at different phases can be uncomfortable – although one cannot avoid experiencing them. Ultimately, we need to move beyond a mechanical process that gives flat results to a deeper understanding, both of the situations we are researching and of the part we play in constructing them.

References

Atkinson, R. (1998) *The Life Story Interview*, Vol. 44. Sage Publications, London.

Atkinson, T. & Claxton, G. (2000) (eds) *The Intuitive Practitioner: On The Value of Not Always Knowing What One is Doing*. Open University Press, Buckingham.

Boud, D. & Walker, D. (1991) 'In the midst of experience: developing a model to aid learners and facilitators'. Paper presented at the *National Conference on Experiential Learning: Empowerment Through Experiential Learning: Exploration of Good Practice*, University of Surrey, Surrey.

Carpenter, C. (2000) Exploring the lived experience of disability. In *Using Qualitative Research* (Hammell, K.W., Carpenter, C. & Dyck, I., eds). Churchill Livingstone, Edinburgh.

Crabtree, B.F. & Miller, W.L. (1999) *Doing Qualitative Research*. Sage Publications, London.

Denshire, S. & Ryan, S. (2001) Using Autobiographical Narrative and Reflection to Link Personal and Professional Domains. In *Professional Practice in Health, Education and the Creative Arts* (Higgs, J. & Titchen, A., eds). Blackwell Science, Oxford.

Fish, D. & Coles, C. (1998) *Developing Professional Judgment in Health Care: Learning Through the Critical Appreciation of Practice*. Butterworth-Heinemann, Oxford.

Fish, D., Twinn, S. & Purr, B. (1991) *Promoting Reflection: The Supervision of Practice in Health Visiting and Initial Teacher Training*. West London Institute Press, London.

Foucault, M. (1994) *The Birth of the Clinic: An Archeology of Medical Perception*. Vintage Books, New York.

Frank, G. (1997) Is there life after categories? Reflexivity in qualitative research. *The Occupational Therapy Journal of Research*, **17**(2), 84–97.

Hunter, E. P. & Blair, S.E.E. (1999) Staff supervision for occupational therapists. *British Journal of Occupational Therapy*, **62**(8), 344–50.

Mason, J. (1996) *Qualitative Researching*. Sage Publications, London.

Mauthner, N. & Doucet, A. (1998) Reflections on a vice centred relational method. In *Feminist Dilemmas in Qualitative Research* (Ribbens, J. & Edwards, R., eds). Sage Publications, London.

Miles, M.B. & Huberman, A.M. (1994) *Qualitative Data Analysis*. Sage Publications, London.

Opie, A. (1992) Qualitative research appropriation of the 'other' and empowerment. *Feminist Review*, **40** (Spring), 53–69.

Pierson, W. (1998) Reflection and nursing education. *Journal of Advanced Nursing*, **27**, 165–70.

Pope, C. & Mays, N. (2000) (eds) *Qualitative Research in Health Care*. BMJ Books, London.

Ryan, S. (2003) *Voices of Recently Graduated Occupational Therapists: Their Practice and Education Stories*. PhD thesis, University of East London.

Schon, D. (1983) *The Reflective Practitioner: How Professionals Think in Action*. Basic Books, New York.

Schon, D. (1987) *Educating the Reflective Practitioner*. Jossey-Bass, San Fransisco.

Smith, S.K. (2000) Sensitive issues in life story research. In *The Researcher Experience in Qualitative Research* (Moch, S.D. & Gates, M.F., eds). Sage Publications, Thousand Oaks, CA.

Watson, J.S. & Wilson, S. (2000) Reading for understanding: methods of reflective practice. *Reflective Practice*, **1**(1), 57–67.

Wellington, B. & Austin, P. (1996) Orientations to reflective practice. *Educational Research*, **38**(3), 307–15.

CHAPTER 5

Navigating multiple research identities: reflexivity in discourse analytic research

Claire Ballinger

Positioning the self: author's story

I am an occupational therapist who for the past twelve years has worked in academic departments of Rehabilitation and Healthcare Professions at the University of Southampton. My initial education in research methods was of a traditional, positivist nature. However, an NHS Research and Development Directorate Research Studentship provided me with an opportunity to fulfil a long-held desire to explore qualitative approaches in more depth. My research interests include perspectives of health, illness and rehabilitation and my work draws on the disciplines of medical sociology, social gerontology and social psychology. The latter has been particularly influential in terms of the methodology adopted for my doctoral work: discourse analysis.

I am excited by the possibilities reflexivity offers for the continual evolution of one's interpretation and position with regard to one's research. Successive drafts of this chapter have, for example, charted my initial discomfort with and attempted resolution of my privileged position as author. However, as a social constructionist who is interested in discursive approaches, I am wary of rhetorical devices used within texts which enable researchers to claim they are 'being reflexive'. I also enjoy attempts to disrupt conventional representations of authorship and forms of writing through humour and irony.

I am currently interested in exploring reflexivity in terms of 'being' rather than 'doing' – that is, as an issue of *subjectivity* rather than method. I am also excited and intrigued by the challenges of reflexivity as a marker of quality in qualitative research.

Introduction

This chapter details my growing insight into the use and value of activities to promote reflexivity. In it, I aim to show, firstly, how reflexivity enabled me to gain an increased awareness of multiple perspectives of health and health events, in particular heightening my sensitivity to the accounts and explanations of service users. Secondly, I hope to demonstrate how the procedures and practices of research impact on data which are produced (and thereby challenging the notion of 'neutral' research practices).

My views on reflexivity took shape as I conducted two empirical research studies. The first focused on accounts of falls and falling in older people provided by occupational therapists and physiotherapists, and older people with fractured hips, in an acute medical care setting (Ballinger & Payne, 2000). The second explored perspectives of risk more broadly, within the context of a day hospital for older people (Ballinger & Payne, 2002). Semi-structured interviews were used in both studies, with the second study additionally employing participant observation and some limited analysis of documentary sources. The methodology underpinning both studies was discourse analysis (Potter & Wetherell, 1987; Parker, 1992). My focus of interest was the constructive potential of talk and writing (described as 'texts'). Specifically, I was probing the common-sense assumptions implicit in texts about the way the world is, the way it works and what it comprises.

Writing a chapter about reflexivity considered through the lens of discourse analysis raises particular issues for me as the author and producer of this account. In discourse analysis the focus is on the construction and function of texts. Here, it is imperative to be reflexive about how one writes about research practices. As Potter (1996) says of his own work, such writings are texts about themselves, showing how particular devices and writing techniques are used in texts to create particular effects.

Within a discursive approach, the act of reflexivity is never complete. During the production of this account, my own position with regard to what I term 'research method' has shifted. In acknowledgement of this, and as a demonstration of reflexivity in action, I have therefore supplemented the main body of the text with footnotes which draw attention to the constructed nature of this chapter as a text.[1]

This chapter is organised in two sections. The first section focuses on the *strategies and practices* I used to enhance reflexivity during my three-year studentship period. Four strategies are described and illustrated with worked examples. In the second section, I attempt to demonstrate some of the *consequences* of these strategies on both the ways in which I carried out the research, and on the development of my analysis.[2]

---

[1] Might this have the effect of unduly fragmenting the text? On the positive side my reflexivity can be witnessed. As with other more experimental forms of writing, such a device offers a positive challenge to the authoritative voice of the writer. It also, rightly I think, emphasises how knowledge is constantly emerging and being constructed.

[2] What forms of writing and representation have I privileged in describing this process and chapter as coherent and structured, rather than being messy and incomplete? This statement minimises both the struggle of writing and the painful process of selecting and prioritising material.

Reflexive strategies and practices

Asking 'difficult' questions

Early on in my research I developed the practice of asking myself 'difficult' questions. The questions were not difficult in that they required detailed or complex answers, but rather that in order to answer them, I required time, often a quiet environment and sometimes additional activities such as reading or discussion to reflect more deeply on what I was doing, and why.

Examples of difficult questions I found useful are:[3]

- What do I understand by 'A'?
- What are the implications of choosing this?
- Why have I done this like B, and not C?
- Why might I have found this?
- Why am I finding this difficult?
- How do I know that I have done this well?
- Can I convince others that this has been done well? If so, how?

A helpful technique in the framing of such questions is to engage in a kind of internalised dialogue, imagining that one's efforts are being critically examined by a variety of different people (such as research participants, research supervisors, academic colleagues, conference delegates, health professionals and potential examiners). This process draws attention to different aspects of one's research: how one might describe it to different people; how to choose and explain theoretical underpinning; the extent to which the work has any practical application.

My status as a full-time research student helped me to focus on the difficult questions as they emerged. With few other demands on my time or tasks in which to take refuge, I realised that in order to proceed I had to address questions which sometimes felt painful, embarrassing, confusing and frustrating. Sometimes posing such a question created a timely and legitimate space in which to refocus on core elements of one's research, in the midst of busy periods such as recruiting participants or analysing data.

The excerpts in Box 5.1 were recorded over several months as I collected data in my initial study. At this time I was having difficulty in making sense of the accounts provided by older service users in response to my interview questions. In contrast, the interviews with therapists seemed much more accessible. The question which stimulated reflexive thinking at this time was 'Why am I finding this so difficult?' The excerpts chart the progress from my initial confusion about

---

[3] How was it that I asked these questions and not others? What can these questions demonstrate about the way I construct the nature and task of 'doing research' and myself as researcher? Am I running the risk of focusing unduly on myself? Or are my questions healthy self-critical challenges?

Box 5.1

13/7/97 EMAIL TO SUPERVISOR
Hi, Sheila
. . . For our meeting on Tuesday, can we discuss my second patient interview, as it raises lots of issues for me about how to handle interviews, and also how justified one is in drawing conclusions from interview data which don't seem to be related particularly to the questions being asked! . . . This would be really helpful as I'm also rethinking my patient questions again (for about the sixth time!) . . . See you on Tuesday, Claire

28/7/97 EXCERPT FROM RESEARCH DIARY
I've now completed 9 therapist interviews and 5 patient interviews. I feel fairly clear that I'm going to consider them separately, that they don't feel the same – this emerged after 2 or 3 patient interviews, in a supervision session with Sheila . . . As yet, I don't have much of a feel about where I'm going with them [patient interviews] . . . The therapist interviews are really starting to be interesting . . . I've really felt the issues growing . . . Interview 7 was electric – it really did start to come together for me then.

18/8/97 EXCERPT FROM RESEARCH DIARY
[written beside a picture of a light bulb, indicating moment of insight!]
It's all part of the same thing – the apportioning of blame, the deciding whose fault it is. Older people attribute the cause of a fall to other people, to themselves, or to fate or bad luck. Therapists tend to blame older people.

17/10/97 EXCERPT FROM RESEARCH DIARY
[on reflecting on a couple of research papers]
. . . some interesting questions surfaced about my work:

(1)   What am I trying to do with my research?
(2)   I guess, how can the people who fall become the subjects of my work if I don't know them? I can only construct them as a therapist, which is to reproduce all the power dynamics . . .
       Hip fractures have increased, leading to alarm in policy and medical circles about cost. At the same time a shift in the way we (i.e. medical community) view events requiring medical care has occurred in that we now view such things as hip fractures as preventable. There is therefore an | interest in falls prevention programmes
(3)   However, older people have not shifted their views in the same way. They view hospital as intimidating, believe there is a moral dimension to the attribution of falls, and that they have to prove that they can cope, that they are being judged.

patient responses to such questions as 'Why do you think the fall happened?' to my growing appreciation of my own role in generating particular sorts of accounts, interpretations and explanations.

Writing a research diary

The value of maintaining a personal research diary throughout the course of one's research – a diary in which one records thoughts and feelings as well as events and process – is well-recognised (Mason, 1996). Such a diary potentially serves many functions: it acts as a chronological record of both sequence of events and development of thinking; it forms a resource in which tentative ideas can be lodged pending further consideration; and it can also serve a cathartic function when one is intellectually puzzled or plain irritated!

For a post-structuralist researcher such as myself for whom texts have a central role as data, the act of reflexively articulating one's thoughts and feelings in written form offers a way of considering one's own subjectivity. Part of one's responsibility as a researcher is then to account for one's own position and subjectivity, and I believe that the writing of a research diary helps to foreground these, making them more accessible both to the researcher and to her readership.

I kept a research dairy over the course of my three-year studentship, which eventually amounted to three full A4 lever-arch files. I kept entries, usually handwritten, in plastic envelopes, each dated and filed in chronological order. This system had the added advantage of providing a means of storing small notes written on odd scraps of paper at times when access to a computer or more formal 'diary' was not available. I also included notes for and on supervision sessions, such as lists of topics or issues which I wanted to discuss. Other contributions such as occasional papers and abstracts were also dated according to the point at which I felt they might be of relevance, and added in chronological order, often accompanied by my commentary detailing why I felt they might be significant or important. This was in addition to a manual index system for papers.

I made additions to the diary as and when I wanted. I rigorously maintained a number of electronic and manual systems for activities such as the monitoring of recruitment to my empirical studies and systematic checking of electronic databases for literature. I therefore wanted my research diary to represent a resource which I did not feel compelled to maintain, but rather where I could engage with intellectual (and personal) challenges connected with my research enterprise when I wished. I enjoyed noting down and reflecting upon the current puzzles, and very often the act of recording these would move my thinking further on.[4]

---

[4] What are the implications of viewing the research diary as a text, or 'data' in itself? Contrast the diary with the thesis resulting from this work. What forms of knowledge do academia recognise? Do I support or challenge academic writing in the way I have constructed this chapter?

The two extracts below in Box 5.2 are from research diary entries written just before the start of my second empirical study, which involved participant observation in a day hospital. My supervisor had suggested that I practise observing and recording everyday occurrences in preparation for this study. The first extract details my confusion, procrastination and uncertainty. The second, recorded a few weeks later, illustrates how my thinking has moved on, following further reading, discussion with my supervisor and reflection. I am able to acknowledge my anxiety, and realise that my questions regarding the process of observation are justified and legitimate.

Box 5.2

15/12/97 FIRST EXCERPT FROM RESEARCH DIARY

I am tired and not feeling well, due to a cold, and have been avoiding doing any observation and reporting, as agreed with Sheila, in preparation for our next meeting together. I start with good intentions, but have been deterred because of the difficulty in finding space after to record what I have seen. I somehow want things to be right before I start, although I know it won't be like that when I start visiting the day hospital. As I become involved in what it is that I am supposed to be observing, I lose my capacity to carry on, and become engaged in the action . . .

5/1/98 SECOND EXCERPT FROM RESEARCH DIARY

I do have quite a lot of anxieties about starting the observation – worries about what to record, how to focus, how to remember, how to avoid going off on a tangent. I remember how acutely uncomfortable I felt on the ward [site of my first study] – where to sit, feeling physically very awkward . . . Yet somehow I feel like I can cope, because these are the very things which will form the basis of the work, the use of me, the reflections on how I feel.

Presenting work to different audiences

Before starting my research, I had been a regular contributor to academic conferences and I was keen to maintain this aspect of my work. Potter and Wetherell (1994, p 64) suggest that 'the regular attempt to make interpretations stand up publicly is a very useful discipline' and I therefore took many opportunities to present both empirical and methodological 'work in progress'. This helped me to reflect on how the quality of my work was perceived by different audiences and also acted as a reflexive strategy to enable me to explore my various identities: occupational therapist, health professional, social science researcher and academic.

As an occupational therapist funded by a research studentship, I viewed fellow health professionals, in particular occupational therapists, as an obvious choice of audience. One current priority of the professions allied to medicine, including occupational therapy, is the establishment of evidence-based practice (Department of Health, 2000). The current political and cultural context in which both health services and health research are practised in the United Kingdom ensures that best outcome and cost effectiveness are never far from the health agenda. While agreeing that these are important priorities, I do not necessarily believe that these should *solely* determine the direction of scholarly inquiry. *Also*, I see the merit in exploring alternative theoretical frameworks through which concepts such as 'evidence' can be understood. In papers prepared for annual conferences of the College of Occupational Therapists, I focused on discourse analysis methodology and theories of risk.

Presenting my work to an audience of occupational therapists helped me to bring issues about my research subjectivity into sharp focus. This process was reinforced when one of my papers was included in the conference section on 'elderly care' rather than in the 'research' stream, where I had expected it to appear. I thought hard about my positioning and responsibilities as a researcher. Was I a therapist interpreting the findings of my research for the benefit of clinical colleagues in order that it might inform their practice and result in better treatment for older people? Was I an academic, introducing new and potentially challenging ideas, stimulating occupational therapists to think about the theoretical basis of their practice? Or was I a social sciences researcher, viewing 'occupational therapy' from without, interested in how occupational therapists construct and legitimate their focus, the boundaries of their practice and their relationships with regard to users of their services? These representations are not mutually exclusive, nor is there a 'right' answer. I have included them to illustrate how the act of representing one's work to others can work reflexively to heighten awareness of one's own subjectivity (or, more precisely, how it is constructed).

Reflecting on difficulties and unexpected findings

This strategy is somewhat different from those already outlined: it details part of the process itself, rather than advocating material ways to stimulate reflexive thinking. However, I include it here in order to highlight areas for inclusion in the critical examination of research practice. Strategies and their consequences are inevitably interconnected. This section illustrates how I developed my own thinking and theorising about researcher identity and position.

While I felt relatively comfortable and confident analysing the transcripts of my interviews with therapists during the first empirical study, I experienced difficulties in making sense of the patient accounts, both during interviewing and as I began analysis. After a while, however, I began to understand how the older people whom I had interviewed were representing themselves in their accounts. While the therapist interviews concurred broadly with my own understandings of falls in older people, the service user accounts seemed to have a protective function, designed to avert possible attributions of carelessness, forgetfulness and frailty. I spent time wondering why this might be, who might be expected to judge in this way, and how my own persona might be implicated in the production of these accounts.

As an occupational therapist with a research training in a broadly positivist tradition, I had little experience of qualitative research generally. Although I had read quite widely around its philosophy, I also had no practical experience of discourse analysis. I knew that preparation and presentation were important when conducting semi-structured interviews, and that ethical considerations also determined procedure. Prior learning and experience led me to believe that I knew how such research interviews could be conducted correctly: that the researcher should behave professionally, dress in a way which was not likely to cause offence, impart the necessary amount of information about the study, gain written consent and generally conduct herself in an efficient and trustworthy manner. Accordingly, I dressed smartly, wore a tag which identified me as a member of university staff and left potential service users information sheets which explained how I had been funded to carry out research which I hoped might improve treatment for people such as themselves. Before interviewing, I carefully worked through consent forms with participants. These asked if they had had the opportunity to discuss the study and ask questions, and assured them that they could decline to participate at any point without this affecting their treatment or care whilst in hospital.

Recruitment of participants was a major practical concern in this first study. The ward from which I was recruiting had a fast throughput of patients, and I was anxious to be able to account for my sample in an academically credible way – for example, ensuring that I had determined the suitability or otherwise of patients to take part in my study before they were discharged or transferred to another ward or hospital. The entry criteria to my study identified that I would include all patients with fractured hips, but exclude those who were confused, could not speak English or who were not well enough to participate. To determine new admissions to and discharges from the ward, I regularly consulted the admissions book, maintained by the ward clerks. Entry criteria for the study were checked with nurses, and I cross-referenced names with medical notes and nurses' card indices kept on the ward. All this seemed to be a relatively unproblematic way of identifying suitable participants.

However, as I reflected on my conduct of the research interviews, it came to me that in many respects I had behaved in the same manner as the health professionals the interview participants had encountered during their hospital stay. I dressed conservatively, wore a badge of identification and accessed patients by initially referring to medical notes and ward staff. Written information about surgical, therapy and ward procedures and consent forms might well have been presented to patients prior to their surgery and on commencement of therapy. The first question of my interview schedule asked patients to tell me about their fall, and the chronological, 'story-like' nature of their responses seemed to suggest that they had done so many times before. I felt in retrospect that they had probably been asked this same question many times by a variety of different health professionals.

These patients had recently experienced a traumatic event, been admitted to hospital as an emergency, received a general anaesthetic and undergone major surgery. By the time of my introduction, they had spent time in several wards and been visited by a number of different health professionals, including doctors, nurses and therapists. Given my apparent ease with the ward routine, it seemed reasonable to assume that service users were responding to me as if I were a health professional. Their future was uncertain, and they were perhaps attempting to retain some control over their destiny by positioning themselves as victims of others' negligence or a random set of circumstances. This explanation is particularly plausible given the lack of privacy in the environment in which they gave their accounts, and the possibility that their accounts might be overheard. My developing interpretation increasingly attended to the service user accounts as representations of competency, lucidity and fitness designed to counter possible negative evaluations (Ballinger & Payne, 2000). By creating time to explore these unexpected interview accounts and their possible functions, I was also able to critically consider my own role in their production.

Some consequences of reflexivity

My reflexive activity in relation to this first study influenced choices made regarding the conduct of my second study. I thought hard about how I had positioned myself as a researcher, and determined that I wanted to 'do it differently' within this second study. I did not believe that my research would be more authentic or valid as a consequence, rejecting these notions as deriving from a realist perspective.[5] However, I wanted to be more actively aware of how I constituted my own position as researcher. I wanted to avoid unknowingly reproducing unequal relations with older health service users in which 'knowledge' (mine) was privileged over 'experience' (theirs). I therefore chose to introduce myself as a student to both staff and service users in the second study (which took place within the context of a day hospital, to which older people were referred for rehabilitation). I dressed more informally, selecting trousers and jumper in preference to skirt and blouse or jacket, and I avoided carrying briefcase, clipboard and sheaths of paper. The same information sheet was provided for service users and staff, in contrast to the different sheets used in the first study,

---

[5] And I want to make my position here clear. What stake do I have in positioning myself in the 'relativist camp'? On what basis do I reject realism? I want to be seen as critical and sophisticated, not naïve and positivist. But are these altogether fair representations?

and I chose not to access any written information about the service or the service users (including medical notes) prior to, or during, data generation.[6]

The initial five weeks of this second study were spent carrying out participant observation, and I chose to physically locate myself with the older service users during this period. The majority spent the large part of their time in the central day room, talking, participating in games, reading the newspaper or sleeping. Most of my periods of observation therefore began here. I accessed additional rooms in the day hospital as service users did; I didn't seek to observe from within the physiotherapy treatment room, for example, until a service user with whom I was talking was invited to attend for physiotherapy. After initially seeking permission both from this woman and her treating physiotherapist, I accompanied her into this room. I attempted to experience the day hospital as far as possible from the perspective of a service user, without prior knowledge about the working of the day hospital, or information about the attending service users.

This was not without its challenges. My early fieldnotes record my sense of self-consciousness and difficulty in simply sitting and observing, in preference to being more active. As a therapist, I saw many opportunities for what would be regarded as therapeutic activities and interactions. Despite this, I deliberately did not pursue or facilitate these, believing such interventions to be at odds with my role as researcher. My relationship with both staff and service users felt ambivalent and unclear. However, it was clear to service users that while I was electing to spend much of my time with them, I was not one of them. For example, I was much younger, and not receiving therapy or medical services. When asked who I was, I stuck with the descriptor 'student', which seemed to imply youth and relative inexperience. However, in response to further questioning about the nature of my studies from one male service user whom I had got to know, I shared the information that I was a postgraduate student and trained health professional. Thus even the self-consciously selected identity of 'student' was ambivalent and open to interpretation.[7]

Summary

Within this chapter I have used specific examples to illustrate how the use of four reflexive practices (asking difficult questions, keeping a research diary, presenting to a variety of audiences and reflecting on difficulties and unexpected findings)

---

[6] At the time of the study I framed my problem in terms of researcher identity and role (e.g. dress, behaviour), but have since come to view it in terms of researcher subjectivity. What might be the implications of this change? Does this mean a different theoretical rationale for my research?
[7] Is it possible to select how one represents one's self, or who one appears to be? Whose perspective is being given pre-eminence in this representation – myself as researcher, or others looking on? What are the implications of this for qualitative research and reflexivity?

facilitated access to different perspectives on health events and challenged 'traditional' research practice conventions. Throughout this chapter, the construction of researcher subjectivity has provided a particular focus through which reflexivity has been explored.

Returning to the issue of representation of reflexivity through a discourse analytic lens, I offer some final questions to consider as part of the ongoing project of constructing researcher subjectivities:

- How do you represent yourself as a researcher?
- How is your discipline or profession implicated in this?
- What assumptions about disciplinary or professional knowledge are reinforced by this?
- How could this be destabilised or challenged?
- Who might benefit from this?
- What do you understand by 'research method'?
- What are the implications of this for the way you are constituted as a researcher?
- What versions of knowledge and 'the truth' are supported within this construction?
- How could this be contested or problematised?
- For whom might this pose a threat?'

Acknowledgements

I would like to thank Kay Price, Centre for Research Into Nursing and Health Care, Division of Health Sciences, University of South Australia for her timely contribution to this chapter.

References

Ballinger, C. & Payne, S. (1997) 'Falls and elderly people – can discourse analysis contribute to understanding?' Paper presented at the *21st Annual Conference College of Occupational Therapists*, Southampton, UK.

Ballinger, C. & Payne, S. (1999) 'An investigation of perceptions of risk in a day hospital'. Paper presented at the *23rd Annual Conference College of Occupational Therapists*, Liverpool, UK.

Ballinger, C. & Payne, S. (2000) Falling from grace or into expert hands? Alternative perspectives about falls in older people. *British Journal of Occupational Therapy*, **63**, 573–79.

Ballinger, C. & Payne, S. (2002) The construction of the risk of falling among and by older people. *Ageing and Society*, **22**, 305–24.

Department of Health (2000) *Meeting the Challenge: A Strategy for the Allied Health Professions*. Department of Health, London.

Mason, J. (1996) *Qualitative Researching*. Sage Publications, London.

Parker, I. (1992) *Discourse Dynamics: Critical Analysis for Social and Individual Psychology*. Routledge, London.

Potter, J. (1996) *Representing Reality: Discourse, Rhetoric and Social Construction*. Sage Publications, London.

Potter, J. & Wetherell, M. (1987) *Discourse and Social Psychology: Beyond Attitudes and Behaviour*. Sage Publications, London.

Potter, J. & Wetherell, M. (1994) Analyzing discourse. In *Analyzing Qualitative Data* (Bryman, A. & Burgess, R.G., eds). Routledge, London.

CHAPTER 6

Developing a critically reflexive position using discourse analysis

David Harper

Positioning the self: author's story

I am a clinical psychologist who practised in the NHS from 1991 to 2000 when I became an academic. I began using Discourse Analysis (DA) in 1990 while researching the social construction of persecutory delusions amongst clinical psychologists and psychiatrists for my postgraduate degree in clinical psychology. I later sought to develop this research by interviewing more people (including users of psychiatric services so diagnosed) and analysing a wider variety of texts, including historical and professional accounts as well as representations circulating in popular culture. My approach to DA has developed over the course of time and is, of course, still developing. I draw on social constructionist and post-structuralist ideas (e.g. deconstruction) but combine these with an approach that has come to be termed critical psychology (e.g. Parker, 1997).

My approach to reflexivity here is structured by three principles. Firstly, since social constructionism is itself a 'social construction' (Burr, 1995), critical attention needs to be focused on my knowledge-making practices and my inscription within historical, professional and cultural texts about paranoia and suspicion. Secondly, I see reflexivity not as an end in itself but rather as a means by which I can be made accountable for my analysis through an explication of my interests and context. I am wary about accounts of reflexivity which rest on simple humanistic notions of being 'open' or 'transparent'. Given the impossibility of 'knowing oneself', a critically reflexive humanism involves more than engaging in 'agonising confessional work' (Parker, 1999, p.31). Moreover, it should be more than a simple listing of the social locations one occupies in order to render them unproblematic. Thirdly, I don't see reflexivity as the only goal of research. If trying to achieve some maximum reflexivity means forsaking other goals, for example, the accessibility of the analysis or the clarification of political and practical implications, I would argue that the balance needs to be redressed. For me, a critical reflection is not a passive contemplative exercise which can paralyse the reader or researcher but instead an 'active rebellious practice that drives individuals into action as they identify the exercise of power that pins them into place and the fault lines for the production of spaces of resistance' (Parker, 1999, p.31).

Introduction

The reflexive aspects of analysis have been largely neglected by discourse analysts. This chapter seeks to address this issue. In particular, I aim to discuss the 'internal workings' of a discourse analysis of interviews about paranoia. I argue that analysis is a struggle after meaning: one involving a wide range of choices and decisions about which there is a need to be explicit. Such choices pose dilemmas for researchers like myself who occupy multiple positions. Negotiating these dilemmas has consequences for the kind of analysis which is produced. Moreover, how can critical researchers negotiate the dilemmas produced by wanting to move from critique and deconstruction to recommending particular interventions in the wider world? Here, I will draw on work from a research project into the social construction of paranoia (Harper, 1994a) which developed ideas from an earlier study (Harper, 1991). The project aimed to identify how paranoia was constructed through delineating some of the assumptions implicit in the notion of paranoid delusions as revealed in professional texts, material from popular culture, and 21 interviews conducted by me: nine with users of mental health services who had been identified by mental health professionals as having experienced paranoid delusions and 12 with professionals who worked with them including psychiatrists, community psychiatric nurses and general practitioners. For the sake of clarity here I will largely focus on the analysis I conducted on the interview material.

The struggle of analysis

The fact that I am focusing on analysis here means that I will not be addressing reflexive aspects of, for example, the formulation of my research questions; the choice of analytic material; the processes of getting the research off the ground, of contacting interviewees, interviewing and transcribing those interviews and so on. Straight away, then, I am demonstrating that writing an account is as much a product of what is *not* attended to and written as it is a product of what *is*. In Discourse Analysis (DA) the activities of 'analysis' and of 'writing up' the research, if not the same, at least overlap. Discourse analyses, like writing in general, are products of choices which the analyst makes within particular contexts with particular aims in mind.

Despite the presence of guiding concerns and questions in the research, such as the questioning of taken-for-granted notions and the revealing of 'hidden' assumptions, I often felt at sea in developing both a theoretical and epistemological position in my analysis of the various textual materials I examined. In their 'ten steps to analyse discourse', Potter and Wetherell (1987) note there is an 'intermission' after transcription of interviews where the researcher is faced with literally hundreds of thousands of words waiting to be transformed into research findings. 'With this thought', they add, 'contentment can easily be transformed into total immobility and panic. Where should one start?' (p.166). They follow this disarming passage with the comment that 'we find it reassuring to begin with some coding' – this rhetorical move unfortunately serves to cover over some of the rich difficulties they note. Hollway (1989) by contrast, comments that making sense of the transcript in terms of the research questions is 'the most harrowing part of all. The more unstructured it is, the greater the anxiety that it is going to be impossible to analyse rigorously' (p.21). My experience seemed to accord more with this latter perspective. Problems in getting interviewees meant that funding for half a day per week off from my full-time day job as a practising NHS clinical psychologist ran out just as I finished transcribing.[1] I spent a good portion of the year following the transcription of interviews in a state of analytic paralysis.

One of the problems was that there seemed too much material to analyse. Would a decision to focus on one aspect rather than another be simply arbitrary? There seemed relatively little in the literature about the process of choosing themes. A relatively routine criticism within DA circles is that themes and discourses do not just 'emerge' from transcripts, rather they are constructed by the analyst. I found both that my codes and categories changed continually and that the connections between them changed too. In the end I made a selection of three analytic themes for the analysis of the interviews. I can justify this selection in terms of the aims and preoccupations of my study, but this does not get away from the fact that *I had to make a choice*.

There is a dual danger here in representing more open-ended approaches to analysis: on the one hand it can be made to seem arbitrary when it was not but also it can be made to seem tidier and more matter-of-fact than it was. There is a need to represent that this analysis was, in Woolgar's (1988) words, a *struggle*. Moreover, the analytic choices I made had certain consequences. Thus I did not focus on other aspects which I could have done, for example the various rhetorical strategies service users and professionals employed in explaining the causes of paranoia. Moreover, looking back, I can see that I used some interview transcripts more than others because they were better examples of some of the themes in which I was interested. Here, too, there were further decisions since I

---

[1] A major material influence on my writing was the actual amount of time I spent on writing and how frequently I was able to write. Other calls on my time (e.g. my employment as a clinical psychologist and my personal life) meant that my writing existed in a particular organisation of time and space and this influenced my writing in a number of ways. On the one hand this helped me to bridge the world of work *in* psychiatry and the world of analysis *of* it. However, it also meant at times that I was prevented from becoming immersed in the analysis of detail, a bit like trying get a good sleep but being constantly wakened.

chose to focus on broader narratives rather than individual cases – Georgaca (1996, 2000), in a similar study, used a more temporally contextualised and individually-focused analytic approach.

I am writing about this experience not to 'confess' my shortcomings as an analyst – I seek only to be a 'good enough' discourse analyst (following Scheper-Hughes' 'good enough' ethnography, 1992, p.28). Rather, I am trying to reveal some of what Figueroa & López (1991) note is lacking in much discourse analytic work: a reflexive attention to the methodological process through which the analysis was produced.

Making the decision-making process explicit: the link between analytic aims and materials

I have noted that I selected three dominant themes from the interview transcripts for further analysis. These were:

- How talk about paranoia was shot through with assumptions about emotions, beliefs and actions (e.g. violence) thought to be driven by those beliefs.
- How notions of plausibility and rationality were drawn on in judging whether beliefs were regarded as paranoid and delusional.
- How psychiatric medication was constructed in the talk of both service users and professionals.

This choice was not entirely arbitrary. It seemed that an analysis of paranoia required an understanding of how it was brought into being and diagnosed (and this rested on how professionals made a judgement of what was and was not delusional); how it was said to be experienced and to affect action; and how it was treated (for all of the service users the primary intervention was psychiatric medication). However, this only seemed obvious after I had begun the analysis. Although following broadly similar practices of categorisation, there were differences in the way my analysis of each of these issues was structured and this seemed to vary according to how I interpreted my general aims in relation to each issue and the shape of the material.

Emotions, beliefs, action and violence

After writing my analysis of texts on the history of paranoia, on how mental health professionals constructed it in their writings and on the way it was represented in popular culture, I began my analysis of the interview transcripts in earnest. I was immediately struck by one thing: my service user interviewees talked a lot about 'being afraid' but this had figured little in the literature I had encountered.

My analysis of this from a discourse analytic viewpoint was helped by the existence of an extensive DA literature on emotion. I then repeatedly read through the interview extracts using a number of analytic questions, e.g. 'What kinds of positions are set up and taken up here?' (Davies & Harré, 1990; Stenner, 1993) or 'What rhetorical strategies and devices are used?' (Edwards & Potter, 1992) or 'To what problems might these responses be solutions?' (Gill, 1995). I selected themes relating to issues such as agency and to binary oppositions such as thought/feeling, mind/body and so on. Again there was a symbiotic link between my interest, the provision of data and the theoretical resources to analyse that data. Simultaneously, I developed theoretical ideas relating to embodiment whilst reading the current literature.

As the analysis developed I realised that it was developing into an examination of how the issue of whether fears were regarded as warranted was influenced by considerations of gender, race, class and so on. I noted that this was linked more to constructions of plausibility and rationality (a second part of my analysis) than to emotion *per se* and so I moved that part of the analysis to this section. I returned to the original categories and realised that an analysis structured around oppositions was more helpful. The themes here, again structured around oppositions, included fear as present/absent, emotion/belief, belief/action and action/violence. The DA literature is replete with renderings of analyses in oppositional form: see, for example, Billig *et al.* (1988). I then worked on these categories to develop a coherent linear narrative structure that followed a reasonably clear theoretical framework.

Discoursing plausibility

For the analysis of the discursive accomplishment of plausibility and rationality, I had already identified a large number of extracts pertaining to this theme and through using similar analytic questions had begun to identify (e.g. in my memos) some rhetorical devices.[2] The choice of analytic category was overdetermined since this issue had interested me during my earlier research on this topic. It was also invited by my general aims since the definition of delusion draws on assumptions about rationality and plausibility. There is an extensive DA literature on the rhetorics of fact construction (see Edwards & Potter, 1992) and this issue was one which all my interviewees touched on. Re-reading the relevant interview extracts, I developed a list of categories and of rhetorical devices used.

---

[2] Discourse analysts use the term rhetorical device to describe ways of talking which are oriented to perform certain functions or have certain effects. Edwards and Potter (1992) outline a number of such devices which speakers may use in constructing accounts as factual, for example 'empiricist accounting' refers to a style or repertoire of discourse common in scientific writing where phenomena are treated as agents in their own right and the subjective investments of investigators and other factors are played down.

As the work progressed, the categories were systematised (i.e. links found between them) and then grouped under similar themes. This process reminded me of other examples of categories in the transcripts and these were then identified. I tried to develop a framework for the analysis so the categories could be grouped to tell a linear story, relevant to plausibility, the central theme of this part of the analysis. As the categories were developed, some extracts did not fit so that categories became further refined. There was also a process of thinning out in which categories which seemed tangential were omitted. For example a category labelled 'miscellaneous' and including sub-categories like 'delusions can be covered up' or 'others may believe in your delusion' was dropped. An initial draft structure was then further clarified.

Mapping medication talk

The construction of professional interventions had hardly been covered in my analysis of the non-interview texts or in my initial categorisation of the interview transcripts. However, it emerged later as I thought about my own and others' neglect of this important topic. As a result I went through the transcripts noting all instances where psychiatric interventions (nearly all relating to medication) were discussed. I also referred to literature on materiality and embodiment and to other research on medication. After this, I categorised the instances. Following a process similar to that adopted elsewhere in my analysis, I developed a reading which had a linear structure but which was more of a mapping-out of the culturally available discourse than the other parts had been. The material was most easily structured along a number of issues, some of which were oppositional in nature. This led me to return to the transcripts, where I found that the other issues could be represented oppositionally too.

Once an overall linear structure had been developed, the criteria for choosing extracts in each part of the analysis of the interview transcripts became clear. Which were the shortest extracts where a particular position was most clearly demonstrated? Which could be understood most easily without having to refer to the rest of that particular interview? Which gave the most diversity in terms of the status of the interviewee (as professional or service user) and in terms of variations on the theme?

My position(s) as a discourse analyst

My analysis was influenced by a variety of factors, external and personal. These included distal factors, for example the new opportunities to conduct critical and qualitative work opened up by the wider crises of legitimacy afflicting psychiatry and medico-scientific discourses generally. This influenced my use of post-structuralist ideas like deconstruction, a social constructionist and qualitative methodology and a critical psychology use of discourse analysis. There were also more proximal factors, for example my personal identification with critical psychology traditions (e.g. Parker *et al.*, 1995), my employment as a mental health professional and my interest in social constructionist approaches to psychological therapy (e.g. Harper, 1995). A consequence of this was my choice of a mental health topic (paranoia), and my interest in analysing non-clinical texts as well as interviews.

The fact that I knew some of my interviewees professionally presented further challenges. Some time after the interviews, but not before I completed my analysis, two of the service user interviewees were referred to me for clinical work. From their point of view I was linguistically, relationally and emotionally part of the psychiatric culture. Despite this, I still thought it possible to be critical of the assumptions implicit in psychiatric accounts. Service user and humanistic psychological accounts (for example, where people talked about their experience of problems or criticised the mental health system) were probably more difficult to unpack because I tended to see them as accurate descriptions of 'reality' which often matched my own views. I felt reluctant to probe the functions of their talk in view of the fact that they were in a powerless position in the system relative to that of myself and other professionals. My role as both practitioner and discourse analyst led to a curious dualism and I began to feel a little like a tight-rope walker (see Sampson (1993) for a description of this metaphor). Barrett (1996) describes his experience of living in two worlds (as a psychiatrist and an anthropologist) as being both an asset and an impediment; his 'familiarity with the world of the psychiatric hospital and its language', he tells us, often made it 'difficult for me to perceive the taken-for-granted assumptions on which that world was built' (p.xvii). He notes how the encouragement of others to maintain a sense of curiosity about what he normally regarded as self-evident enabled him to make use of his cultural competence in an analytic way. For me, too, discussions with my supervisor, reading others' work, writing at home (rather than at my clinical workplace), writing for publication (and thus getting feedback from independent reviewers) and discussions with others at conferences and elsewhere helped the process. As Stenner & Stainton-Rogers (1998) note, interpretation draws on the researcher's theoretically and culturally embedded expectations but this need not preclude the possibility that one can be surprised in the process of analysis.

There were other tensions and dilemmas. Burman & Parker (1993) note the ethical issues involved in interpreting the words of others. Stainton-Rogers (1991) comments that 'in order to weave my story, I must inevitably do violence to the ideas and understandings as they were originally expressed' (p.10). As I worked on my analysis, I asked such questions as: 'Have I been symmetrical, equally respectful and non-blaming of all participants?' and 'Has there been any creeping intentionalism on my part?' Often, early drafts showed that there had been. For example, one section of my analysis of talk about medication was concerned with how the interviewees accounted for the apparent failure of medication. My initial reading emphasised what interviewees might achieve by giving accounts which absolved the medication or professionals of responsibility.[3] However, I came to see that psychiatric discourse is hegemonic in that I, too, was located in this way of talking. It is a danger of discourse analytic work that it can locate agency either in the person or in complexes of institutional power relations (Cobb, 1994). However, a discursive approach may equally well provide an analysis that avoids falling into such dualist traps by taking a both/and rather than an either/or position. The acts of an individual are social in origin and have social consequences (and vice versa).

It can also be easy for researchers to be critical of individuals, especially those seen to be in positions of authority. I sought to ensure a number of counterbalances to avoid my analysis being seen as implied criticism of individuals. Firstly, I purposely wrote the analysis in such a way that the focus was on the talk and its effects, regardless of the 'motivations' of any individual speaker: I did not want to engage in any psychological interpretations of their verbal and other behaviour. Secondly, I aimed to be scrupulous in not revealing the identities of the participants. Thirdly, I included myself in the analysis and demonstrated that the discussion was not something simply engaged in by others.

There is a danger when researchers lose their reflexivity and see themselves as lying outside the arena of discourse. One of the results of the research for me was the revelation that *I, too, was located within psychiatric discourse.* Rather than seeing positioning as something others were doing, I recognised that I was also implicated. This could be seen in a number of ways: from the words and terms that I used in the interviews (e.g. 'diagnosis', 'paranoia'), to the fact that, on some occasions, I found the beliefs of some participants to be extremely implausible. Part of my analysis of plausibility focused on an extract from an interview with a current user of psychiatric services and attempted to track a breakdown in the discursive accomplishment of plausibility between us. This, I found, was an interactional process: the breakdown occurred both because of what was said by the interviewee and because of the particular cultural assumptions and expectations I brought to the interview. I was not claiming to write about paranoia as something only others do – the traditional research focus – but as a form of discourse – and a position in discourse – that everyone, myself included, uses.

Analysis and participant validation

I have examined some of the ways my reflexivity influences analysis. In particular, I have highlighted how analysis involves choices and how those choices

---

[3] See Harper (1999b) for more on this. Interestingly, Lucy Johnstone's (2000) discussion of this work alludes to the purpose rather than the effects of such strategies.

have consequences. Of course, one choice is about what kind of analysis one undertakes and this has implications for whether or not research will be fed back to research participants. Burr (1995), for example, has argued for participants' validation of a researcher's account as a criterion for quality control, though Sherrard (1991) comments that such validation rarely happens. Smith (1995) notes that whether to do this and if so, how, depends on the aim of the research project. If one is attempting to produce an account that fits with interviewees' experience (as ethnomethodologists or phenomenologists might seek to do) or which might even be useful to them as a description, then feeding back is essential. But what if this is not the aim of the research?

In some previous research I conducted on the theme of paranoia, one of my psychologist interviewees was invited to write a commentary on one of the reports (Garety, 1994). Among other things, she was concerned that I was not describing the views I was getting in enough detail.[4] Nowadays I would be much more explicit with interviewees about what form the analysis would take. However, when I was interviewing for that earlier project (1990–91) and even for the next project (1993–94) it would have been difficult to be explicit since I was not sure myself how the analysis would develop.

A further difficulty with validation is what to do when interviewees reach views on the analyst very different from those of the analyst him- or herself. Those in more powerful positions might feel threatened by an account which revealed the extent of that power and how it was deployed (Kitzinger & Wilkinson, 1997). Coyle (1995) identifies another problem: given the post-structuralist assumption that meaning is not fixed, language use might have consequences that the speaker did not intend. For example, the speaker might invoke discourses and ideologies of which they were not actually aware.

My aims were not ethnomethodological and I was not aiming to represent how the participants saw the situation, so I did not feed my analysis back to my participants. There were practical and ethical constraints, too. For example, 'which "analysis" would I feed back?', 'Would I expect participants to read an academic thesis?' Moreover, when I originally gained consent I had not asked whether participants would be willing to allow their accounts to be read by other interviewees. The issue of participant validation seemed to present a dual danger. On the one hand, it struck me as somewhat arrogant to assume that the research was so important to the participants that they needed to see my account in order not to feel disempowered. On the other hand, it seemed premature to assume that the research was not important and would not have any effect on the participants.

---

[4] There were also issues about the amount of data I included which was constrained by reviewers' requirements that I justify my epistemological and methodological position and explain the theory and procedure of DA since such work was far from common in mental health journals at that time.

In the end, pragmatic considerations seemed to win the day. I decided I would see some post-research discussion as important if the research had taken up a good deal of the participant's time: it seemed appropriate to explain my analyses and seek their views. Where, however, I had spent less than an hour with interviewees, I decided against testing participants' patience and goodwill by seeking to take up even more of their time. The research, while important to me, might not be so to them.

As Smith (1994) notes, there are practical constraints on the ability to be reflexive. As in his case, I had others to interview, a thesis to complete and, in addition, a day job. Of course, the situation might be different in the case of an action research project formulated by service users; here, discussing findings with participants would be a central part of the project since they would be its commissioners. Even now, some time after finishing my analysis, I feel some uneasiness at the absence of participant validation for my study, and wonder whether this had any effects on my analysis. For example, might this lack of accountability have led me to be too 'free' in interpreting the words of others? A further problem was the gap of nearly six years between the original interviews (1993–94) and the finishing of the subsequent analysis (1999). Such a gap can cause difficulties for subsequent attempts to contact participants since 'the trail seems cold, one fears they will hardly remember' (Harper, 1998).

Telling the story straight: creating a linear narrative

My writing was also influenced by the need to develop a coherent, consistent and linear argument, to tell a particular story. To this end, I marshalled evidence and sought to make a case. Those reading my research, then, need to keep an eye on the rhetorical strategies (e.g. of plausibility and persuasiveness) used to produce linearity. Stainton-Rogers (1991) notes that the implication of telling a story is that it is 'a distorted and partial version that I have deliberately constructed for you in a particular way, for particular reasons' (p.10). Scheper-Hughes (1992) comments that what emerges from writing is 'highly subjective, partial, and fragmentary' (1992, p.xii). Stainton-Rogers suggests that she is not telling it 'like it is' but rather saying 'look at it this way' (p.10). In the process, many things are left out; in my own case, I have focused on only a narrow range.

The production of linear accounts raises certain dilemmas. One is continually tempted to step back from the writing and reflect on the written account, or go off at apparent tangents and make a connection elsewhere. What is lost for the sake of developing a linear logical argument? There is, of course, never a definitive 'finished' version of an analysis. Rather, analyses are oriented to a particular purpose (reporting to a grant-awarding body, completing a PhD thesis, securing publication in a journal and so on). They are also, to some extent at least, provisional since they are the products of a continual iterative cycling between reading and writing. This process is punctuated by practical requirements like the writing of a thesis. My analysis was a snapshot of something that is actually dynamic and as versions of it are rewritten (like this chapter) they are also revised. The published accounts (Harper, 1992, 1994) differed from the original thesis (Harper, 1991) for a number of reasons: the thesis was written to a course deadline whereas more time could be devoted to the articles, which were also influenced by the need to write self-contained accounts.

As well as a wish to be reflexively aware, another of my aims was to develop the practical implications of my research. I also wanted it to be accessible to different audiences. For me, political and ethical ends are more important than theoretical 'purity' (though, of course, I am constructing an opposition here). This is easier to say than to practise, since theories, values and politics are continually in conflict. A more dialectical and pragmatic approach might be to acknowledge that different positions in discourse are not right or wrong but simply enable certain possibilities of thought and action together with certain dangers and constraints.

Reflexivity and the wider world: implications and interventions

Critics of reflexivity, or rather an overemphasis on it, note that it can lead to a paralysis (Burman & Parker, 1993). One could argue that proper reflection on one's research should include consideration of its implications for the wider world. The final part of my analysis included a discussion of some of the tensions and dilemmas in going beyond an analysis of discourse to outline implications for intervention.[5] I focused not only on the minutiae of 'my findings' about paranoia but also on some broader consequences of the research. This was because I did not want these suggestions to be framed by a concept already constructed within a dominant psychiatric discourse. Danziger (1997) has noted a danger in using constructionism as a form of critique, since the use of traditional categories (like 'paranoia') in critical accounts serves to perpetuate the dominant discourse – the 'old wine, new bottles' problem.

The idea of suggesting implications which cut across such categories is, of course, an intervention in itself. One problem is that one could draw such implications without having done the research – in other words, that there is no link between doing the study and drawing the implications. There are two responses to this. Firstly, interventions do not necessarily have their origin in academic research in any case. Secondly, implications need to have specificity,

---

[5] There is debate about whether making recommendations based on such research is contradictory, a form of 'ontological gerrymandering' – see Harper (1999b) for an account of my position on this.

and empirical studies can bring this and offer insights that might otherwise seem counter-intuitive and surprising. My aim was, in the light of all the possible interventions one could make, to determine which were the 'better' ones and which were most consistent with my conclusions.

It would be a mistake to assume that DA research is straightforwardly applicable. There are a number of problems: for instance, what constitutes 'research' and what constitutes 'research findings'? Moreover, what counts as an 'intervention'? These questions seem particularly pertinent at the end of a discourse analysis where there are no summary statistics of 'findings' and where attempts to give a broad sweep might lead to excessively vague generalisations or the banal restatement of interview transcripts. I found it helpful to focus on particular target groups: academic researchers in psychiatry and allied fields like nursing, social work and clinical psychology, practitioners in those fields; the wider group of practitioners involved in providing psychotherapy and counselling; users of mental health services and their relatives and friends. I asked what might be of interest or use to them, and what might be the most influential medium of communication for each group.

Summary

Interventions do not flow directly from research, rather the use of these ideas is a matter of practical and reflexive engagement. Even if forms of DA and deconstruction are not used explicitly they may still *inform* interventions. The relationship between 'theory' and 'practice' needs to be seen as less linear and separate but, rather as dialectical, recursive and reflexive. Reflection on practice is theorising and theorising is itself a practice.

Acknowledgements

I would like to thank Gary Brown, Erica Burman, Genie Georgaca, Ian Parker, Mark Stowell-Smith and Carla Willig for making helpful comments on an earlier version of this chapter. I'm also grateful to a number of trainee clinical psychologists, mainly on the Doctoral Degree in Clinical Psychology at the University of East London, for giving valuable encouragement.

REFERENCES

Barrett, R.J. (1996) *The Psychiatric Team and the Social Definition of Schizophrenia: An Anthropological Study of Person and Illness*. Cambridge University Press, Cambridge.

Billig, M., Condor, S., Edwards, D., Gane, M., Middleton, D. & Radley, A. (1988) *Ideological Dilemmas: A Social Psychology of Everyday Thinking*. Sage Publications, London.

Bola, M., Drew, C., Gill, R., Harding, S., King, E. & Seu, B. (1998) Representing ourselves and representing others: a response. *Feminism & Psychology*, 8, 105–10.

Burman, E. & Parker, I. (eds) (1993) *Discourse Analytic Research: Repertoires and Readings of Texts in Action*. Routledge, London.

Burr, V. (1995) *An Introduction to Social Constructionism*. Routledge, London.

Cobb, S. (1994) A critique of critical discourse analysis: deconstructing and reconstructing the role of intention. *Communication Theory*, 4, 132–52.

Coyle, A. (1995) Discourse analysis. In *Research Methods in Psychology* (Breakwell, G.M., Hammond, S. & Fife-Shaw, C., eds). Sage Publications, London.

Danziger, K. (1997) The varieties of social construction. *Theory & Psychology*, 7, 399–416.

Davies, B. & Harré, R. (1990) Positioning: The discursive production of selves. *Journal for the Theory of Social Behaviour*, 20, 43–63.

Edwards, D. & Potter, J. (1992) *Discursive Psychology*. Sage Publications, London.

Figueroa, H. & López, M. (1991) 'Commentary on discourse analysis workshop/conference'. Paper for *Second Discourse Analysis Workshop/Conference*, Manchester Polytechnic, July.

Fox, D. & Prilleltensky, I. (eds) (1997) *Critical Psychology: An Introduction*. Sage Publications, London.

Garety, P.A. (1994) Construction of 'paranoia': does Harper enable voices other than his own to be heard? *British Journal of Medical Psychology*, 67, 145–46.

Georgaca, E. (1996) *Exploring 'Psychotic Discourse': The Construction and Negotiation of Reality and Subjectivity in Language*. Unpublished PhD thesis, Manchester Metropolitan University.

Georgaca, E. (2000) Reality and discourse: A critical analysis of the category of 'delusions'. *British Journal of Medical Psychology*, 73, 227–42.

Gill, R. (1995) Relativism, reflexivity and politics: interrogating discourse analysis from a feminist perspective. In *Feminism & Discourse* (Wilkinson, S. & Kitzinger, C., eds). Sage Publications, London.

Harper, D.J. (1991) *'Just Because I'm Paranoid Doesn't Mean They're Not Out to Get Me': A Discourse Analytic Approach to 'Paranoia'*. Unpublished M. Clin. Psychol. thesis, Department of Clinical Psychology, University of Liverpool.

Harper, D.J. (1992) Defining delusion and the serving of professional interests: the case of 'paranoia'. *British Journal of Medical Psychology*, 65, 357–69.

Harper, D.J. (1994) The professional construction of 'paranoia' and the discursive use of diagnostic criteria. *British Journal of Medical Psychology*, 67, 131–43.

Harper, D.J. (1995) Discourse analysis and 'mental health'. *Journal of Mental Health*, 4, 347–57.

Harper, D. (1998) Discourse analysis and psychiatric medication. *Clinical Psychology Forum*, 114, 19–21.

Harper, D.J. (1999a) *Deconstructing Paranoia: An Analysis of the Discourses Associated with the Concept of Paranoid Delusion*. Unpublished PhD thesis, Department of Psychology & Speech Pathology, Manchester Metropolitan University.

Harper, D. (1999b) Tablet talk and depot discourse: discourse analysis and psychiatric medication. In *Applied Discourse Analysis: Social and Psychological Interventions*. (Willig, W., ed.). Open University Press, Buckingham.

Harper, D. (2002a) The tyranny of expert language. *Open Mind*, **113**, 8–9.

Harper, D. (2002b) When the drugs don't work. *Open Mind*, **114**, 8.

Harper, D. (in press) Moving beyond the tyranny of expert language. *Open Mind*.

Henwood, K.L. & Pidgeon, N.F. (1992) Qualitative research and psychological theorizing. *British Journal of Psychology*, **83**, 97–111.

Hollway, W. (1989) *Subjectivity and Method in Psychology: Gender, Meaning and Science*. Sage Publications, London.

Johnstone, L. (2000) *Users and Abusers of Psychiatry*, 2nd edn. Routledge, London.

Kitzinger, C. & Wilkinson, S. (1997) Validating women's experience? Dilemmas in feminist research. *Feminism & Psychology*, 7, 566–74.

Parker, I. (1992) *Discourse Dynamics: Critical Analysis for Social and Individual Psychology*. Routledge, London.

Parker, I. (1994) Reflexive research and the grounding of analysis: social psychology and the psy-complex. *Journal of Community & Applied Social Psychology*, **4**, 239–52.

Parker, I. (1997) Discursive psychology. In *Critical Psychology: An Introduction* (Fox, D. & Prilleltensky, I., eds). Sage Publications, London.

Parker, I. (1999) Critical reflexive humanism and critical constructionist psychology. In *Social Constructionist Psychology: A Critical Analysis of Theory and Practice* (Nightingale, D.J. & Cromby, J., eds). Open University Press, Buckingham.

Parker, I., Georgaca, E., Harper, D., McLaughlin, T. & Stowell-Smith, M. (1995) *Deconstructing Psychopathology*. Sage Publications, London.

Potter, J. & Wetherell, M. (1987) *Discourse and Social Psychology: Beyond Attitudes and Behaviour*. Sage Publications, London.

Ricoeur, P. (1970) *Freud and Philosophy: An Essay on Interpretation*. Yale University Press, London.

Rose, N. (1989) *Governing the Soul: The Shaping of the Private Self*. Routledge, London.

Sampson, E.E. (1993) Identity politics: challenges to psychology's understanding. *American Psychologist*, **48**, 1219–30.

Scheper-Hughes, N. (1992) *Death Without Weeping: The Violence of Everyday Life in Brazil*. University of California Press, Berkeley.

Sherrard, C. (1991) Developing discourse analysis. *Journal of General Psychology*, **118**, 171–79.

Smith, J.A. (1994) Towards reflexive practice: engaging participants as co-researchers or co-analysts in psychological inquiry. *Journal of Community & Applied Social Psychology*, 4, 253–60.

Smith, J.A. (1995) Semi-structured interviewing. In *Rethinking Methods in Psychology* (Smith, J.A., Harré, R. & Van Langenhove, L., eds). Sage Publications, London.

Stainton-Rogers, W. (1991) *Explaining Health and Illness: An Exploration of Diversity*. Harvester Wheatsheaf, London.

Stenner, P. (1993) Discoursing jealousy. In *Discourse Analytic Research: Repertoires and Readings of Texts in Action* (Burman, E. & Parker, I., eds). Routledge, London.

Stenner, P. & Stainton-Rogers, R. (1998) Jealousy as a manifold of divergent understandings: a Q methodological investigation. *European Journal of Social Psychology*, **28**, 71–94.

Walkup, J. (1994) Commentary on Harper, 'The professional construction of paranoia and the discursive use of diagnostic criteria'. *British Journal of Medical Psychology*, **67**, 147–51.

Willig, C. (ed.) (1999a) *Applied Discourse Analysis: Social and Psychological Interventions*. Open University Press, Buckingham.

Willig, C. (1999b) Beyond appearances: A critical realist approach to social constructionist work. In *Social Constructionist Psychology: A Critical Analysis of Theory and Practice* (Nightingale, D.J. & Cromby, J., eds). Open University Press, Buckingham.

Woolgar, S. (1988) Reflexion on Potter. In *Knowledge and Reflexivity: New Frontiers in the Sociology of Knowledge* (Woolgar, S., ed.). Sage Publications, London.

CHAPTER 7

Reflexivity as presence: a journey of self-inquiry

Gweneth Doane

Positioning the self: author's story

As a person who professionally lives and enacts the roles of psychologist, nurse, researcher and university professor, I have gradually come to understand how vital reflexivity is to my everyday work. And, as I have become aware of how important reflexivity is to my work I have felt the need to develop more knowledge about it. I have found myself wanting to know and experience reflexivity – both as an academic and as a deeply-engaged person who seeks to involve herself with others.

Although I have not found any label that captures the philosophical or theoretical perspective I bring to my work, I share many of the beliefs and goals of the pragmatist philosophers such as John Dewey and Richard Rorty. Like these pragmatists, my overall aim as a person-researcher is to become ever more sensitive to people. I seek to take people's experiences into account, even more than I have previously. My aspirations as a researcher are similar to Rorty's (1989) description of pragmatists who are inspired by the hope 'to make the best selves for ourselves that we can' (p. 80). As a researcher I have, in essence, looked for ways to be the best I can be, in terms of being sensitive to people and their experiences.

The chapter in this book offers an example of how I have come to understand and live reflexivity as 'consciousness-without-content'. Although I use suffering to exemplify the power of such reflexivity, I believe it offers a way of accessing knowledge of *any human experience*. As I have lived and developed my ability to be relationally and reflexively present with people, and have consciously practised ongoing self-inquiry, my experiences and work as a researcher have been greatly enriched.

Introduction

Although there is no doubt that reflexivity can aid the research process and offer avenues into important spheres of knowledge, in this chapter I discuss a realm of human experience that existing reflexive practices, at least the ones I have read about, do not seem to access.

I begin my discussion by briefly relating an experience that served to inspire my thinking about reflexivity. Next, I provide a brief piece of writing from a process of self-inquiry that helped me to clarify my thoughts. And, finally, I invite you, the reader, to consider a further possibility for reflexivity – one that involves an attentive dwelling, a deep relational presencing through which it is possible to access another mode of consciousness and thus realm of knowledge.

A conversation

The experience that sparked further contemplation of reflexivity was a presentation I attended during a research conference. The presentation focused on reflexivity and its relevance for helping researchers manage the difficulty they may experience when they hear deeply moving stories of pain and suffering. The following is a quote from the actual paper that was presented:

> 'In the face of such anxiety-provoking situations, the researcher necessarily closes off, necessarily fails to listen, and fails to be receptive, at least at times. The question should not be how does one remain open, as if one could attain such a state continuously, but how can one maintain some degree of openness even as one also, in part, turns away' (Dahlberg & Halling, 2000).

The presenters provided an opportunity for an in-depth discussion of their ideas. Although it is impossible to summarise all that was said during that discussion, it seemed to me (as a listener-participant) that two underlying assumptions were shaping the conversation. First, it was assumed that relating to people who are suffering is a difficult thing that at times can be overwhelming. Different members of the group provided concrete examples of experiences they had had where they felt distress and despair as they listened to participants recount painful experiences. The second assumption that seemed to guide the discussion was that the nexus of control for managing the feelings that arose through that difficulty was situated with the researcher. That is, researchers were seen as responsible for dealing with the pain experienced and ensuring their subjective experience did not inadvertently affect the inquiry. And *reflexivity* was the process researchers could use to achieve this. Interestingly, this closing off approach has been highlighted and critiqued by feminist researchers (Stanley & Wise, 1983), yet it seems that it still dominates and directs researchers in many situations.

As I sat listening to the discussion I found myself greatly perturbed by what was seemingly known by the group – that suffering required a turning away and that reflexivity was a process that could help researchers manage their subjectivity and their pain. Although I could not actually name what my discomfort was, my bodily response (the turmoil in my stomach and the squirming feeling I had as I sat in my chair) told me that this 'knowledge' was inconsistent with my experience of suffering and/or how I live reflexivity when relating to suffering.

I left the conference feeling somewhat muddled and confused, still pondering the idea that it was necessary to 'close off' in order to do good research. As I thought about it more, it seemed to me that closing off implied a separateness of self and life world. The language of openness and of turning away seemed to imply that people were separate from the 'other', to the point that they could actually choose to be relating or not. As I thought about this, I realised that part of my discomfort was due to the assumptions I hold about self and subjectivity. Since I think of self as a reality drawn forth in the relational moment (McNamee, 1996; McNamee & Gergen, 1999) – and believe we are, in essence, relational beings – it does not seem possible to me to turn away, to separate ourselves from what is happening. We are not separate from others and therefore do not have the choice to be unaffected. For example, when I felt discomfort with the conversation at the conference I could have cognitively decided not to think about it and chosen to focus my conscious attention on something else. However, I *know* my experience to be embodied. Whether I am consciously remaining open or consciously closing off, I experience the text as *continuing to live in me*, having material effects on my body, on my self, and on my experience.

An inquiry into suffering

As I became clearer about how my assumptions of a relational self were triggering a lot of my discomfort, the researcher in me began to wonder if an individualist conceptualisation of self and the experience of separateness that arose from that conceptualisation might not be giving rise to, or at least contributing to, the difficulty the researchers experienced as they listened to people's stories of pain and suffering. I thought about the experiences some of the researchers shared during the conference discussion and their descriptions of what it had been like for them to listen to painful stories. This reflection sparked a desire to learn more about my own experience of suffering and to know more about how *I* was when relating to suffering. I decided to undertake a self inquiry – re-entering and inquiring into my own experiences of coming face-to-face with suffering. This inquiry involved keeping a journal in which to write through my thinking as well as meditatively re-entering and reliving my experiences in an embodied way.

During this inquiry process two experiences immediately came to the forefront of my awareness. The first was an experience many years ago when I was a young nurse working in an Intensive Care Unit. The second, an experience a few years later, occurred after the sudden death of my brother. The following (see Box 7.1) is some of my writing during the self-inquiry into those experiences. I share it with you in an effort to invite you into my thinking and illuminate, at least in part, how the questions regarding reflexivity have arisen within me.

As an Intensive Care Unit nurse I had considered myself well-armed in my

---

Box 7.1 Experience One: Powerlessness in the Intensive Care Unit

ICU is quiet, but the hospital is overflowing. As I come on duty I am told that one of my patients is in our unit temporarily because she needs a private room. She is a young woman in her late 20s who has just been told she has terminal cancer. As I listen to the report a number of thoughts and feelings flood through me. She's only a few years older than me! What must she be going through? I have never really looked after anyone who is dying. I mean, sure lots of people die in our unit, but they are in our unit because we are trying to stop them from dying – what do I do for someone who is here because she is dying?

I head out of the office and into the young woman's room. I say hello and introduce myself. She just turns around and looks at me. I find myself asking how she is (inside I am berating myself 'How can you ask such an inadequate question?!'). She just turns over in her bed. I check her intravenous and flee – I tell myself that my other patient might need me. A little while later I go back in to check on the young woman. As I enter the room I hear her crying. I stand there feeling totally inadequate. 'What should I say? What if I say the wrong thing?' I do my check. I don't acknowledge her tears and once again I flee.

---

technical know-how, yet here was a situation where my armour came up short. My solid grounding in technological know-how was no foundation for relating to another's suffering. My understanding of the difficulty I experienced was shaped by my existing assumptions and beliefs about suffering. As in a *palimpsest* (Davies, 1993), my new understandings were written over older writings on an already existing parchment. I vividly remember believing there was a 'right' thing to say and my realisation that I didn't know it, was interpreted by me as a lack of skill. This interpretation actually played an important part in my decision to return to university. My desire was to become more skilful at communicating so I would not be ill-equipped to care in future situations. Overall, the story I created of my experience was one of being faced with human suffering, having no available method for treating it, and needing to develop ways and 'know-how' for the future.

As my story reveals, suffering is something that 'humbles us, brings us up short, stops us in our tracks, something surpassing which inspires a mix of fear and awe and admiration, something which both strikes us down and draws us near' (Caputo, 1987, p. 275). I *re-member* that feeling of being stopped in my tracks, my fear of the young woman's suffering and the powerlessness I feel in my inability to change it. I *re-member* how her suffering sparks a deep suffering of my own. I *re-member* how, even though I flee from her physical presence, her suffering (and my own) goes with me.

I vividly re-member how revelatory it was in the second experience to have someone simply be with me without trying to ease my pain. As I try to write

Box 7.2 Experience Two: The Power of Relational Presence

As I hang up from my friend who has phoned to offer her condolences the tears begin to flow and another wave of grief sweeps over me. Taking my box of Kleenex I sit down on the couch to ride the wave and be in my grief. After a few minutes I become aware of Adrian (my four-year-old son) standing in front of me. On his face is an expression of concern as he asks me what is wrong. 'I'm feeling very sad about Uncle Gary so I'm just letting the sadness come out for awhile', I reply. With that he nods and I watch as he walks off into the family room. A minute later he returns carrying his most precious teddy. Without saying a word he hands me his teddy, crawls up on my lap, and just sits with his arms wrapped around me. After a while, as the wave of grief gradually sweeps away, I smile down at him and ask if he would like me to read him a book. He nods, smiles, and goes off to choose some books.

about that experience (see Box 7.2) the image of standing under a waterfall emerges. Standing alone under the water that is coming with torrential force, it is as if I may well be knocked over by the strength of the water. As my son joins me, that feeling somehow changes. Together we are able to support each other even though the water continues to rush down. What is so profound is where my son is putting his focus and energy. He wraps his arms around me and puts his energy into just being (relationally) with me. He in no way attempts to lessen the force of the water. He does not try to help me out of the waterfall or look for ways to shelter me or himself from the force of the downpour. Gradually, I realise I am no longer focusing on the waterfall, but on the feeling of being relationally with him. In a gestalt, the pain and fear of the waterfall moves to the background and the relational flow that my son and I are living moves to the foreground.

Re-entering these experiences I see how they have profoundly shaped my understanding of human suffering and the way I am when relating with people who are experiencing pain in their lives. I see how I have come to relationally enter the abyss of human suffering with intentionality and willingness to be in the abyss, to honour and live the difficulty that is there. Similarly to Caputo's (1987) description, I have taken the occasion to be 'instructed by the abyss, to let the abyss be, to let it play itself out, not in a passive gesture of surrender to destruction but in the sense of what Heidegger calls openness to the mystery' (p. 278). Csikszentmihalyi's (1993) flow experience comes to mind. I willingly enter into the relational flow of the abyss and to a place of non-action. By joining with the flow – by being in the abyss – I am able to move beyond breaking down or detachment from suffering.

Some important unlearning

Through my self-inquiry, I realise I have been living some important 'unlearning' over the past many years. My personal experiences of suffering and the relational experiences I have had as a psychologist and nurse have helped me to unlearn some socially constructed knowledge and skills that have constrained my ability to enter the relational realm. The unlearning of these skills reawakened my spontaneous human capacity for embodied presence to another. The unlearning was similar to Varela *et al.*'s (1993) analogy of being born 'already knowing how to play the violin and practising with great exertion only to remove the habits that prevented one from displaying that virtuosity' (p. 251).

Through my unlearning, the way I live the reflexive process has also been transformed. Like my young son, I now extend myself to be self-abandonedly immersed in relationship. Forgetting my-*self* I am able to eclipse the grasping and floundering that emerges from my own meaning constructions and the opposi-tional schemes they give rise to. Experience is no longer good or bad, privileged or unprivileged, hopeful or unhopeful. Rather, it just is.

This self-abandonment does not mean lack of consciousness; rather my energy is concentrated on self–other relations as opposed to the separateness of self, other and action (Paterson & Zderad, 1976). Consciousness moves beyond some realm of interiority or self-awareness and involves a reaching out and intending (Greene, 1995). I no longer focus on what is happening for me or for the other person(s). Moving beyond the intersubjectivity of two separate beings, attention is on the life that is welling up and flowing through our togetherness in the moment. May's (1982) description of unitary experiences speaks to the form of consciousness I am attempting to describe. According to May, in unitary experiences there is no separateness between self and other. In unitary experi-ences there is consciousness-without-content:

> 'The idea of experience or perception without the presence of the experiencer or perceiver is untenable in Western thought . . . Even so, it is just as true that consciousness-without-content contains no perception, no experience, no anything. And yet it is not a state of nothingness. Everything is there, immediately present and absolutely clear. Perception occurs, but without anything being perceived and without anyone perceiving' (May, 1982, p. 45).

Although everything is there and immediately present, in consciousness-with-out-content there is no action or reaction that would in any way separate the observer from the observed (May, 1982). May describes that it is as though one moves directly into the immediate world just-as-it-is. As such, the opportunity to experience another realm of knowing and understanding is created.

Reconstituting reflexivity

Although the ideas of presencing and relationship are not new to the reflexivity literature, the way these processes are currently discussed has the ring of an alienated mode of consciousness which sees the knower as separate from the known (Heshusius, 1994). Regardless of whether reflexivity is conceptualised as introspection, intersubjective reflection, mutual collaboration, social critique or discursive deconstruction (Finlay, 2002), the process includes acts of observation, analysis, and interpretation. The researcher is in an active mode of consciousness that requires an act of stepping back. That is, the researcher's consciousness moves back and forth between self and other in order to observe and interpret. This active mode and the self-consciousness it requires may actually create a separateness between the researcher and the researched. Although the intersubjective process implies a participatory mode of relationship and consciousness, this managed form of subjectivity and participation seems similar to a subtle version of empiricist objectivity (Heshusius, 1994).

However, reflexivity-as-presence, as *consciousness-without-content*, moves the reflexive process beyond the business (and bus-i-ness) of thinking and acting and beyond the level of the researcher. As the researcher no longer seeks to observe or interpret, he or she does not need to step back from the inquiry process and/or from research participants. Reflexivity-as-presence is not a methodology with methodological strategies but rather a mode of consciousness involving in-active action (Weil, 1992). The mode of consciousness requires that the researcher move beyond self-awareness and beyond the act of interpreting. It involves the ability to let go of preoccupations with self and to be in a place of complete attention. It requires being with others in a way that leads to a heightened feeling of aliveness and awareness (Heshusius, 1994). Reflexivity-as-presence does not provide another map for the reflexive process. Rather, it offers a possibility for moving beyond ourselves and our current ways of knowing by reflexively shifting our focus and intent.

Heshusius (1994) has discussed a similar process to the one I have been attempting to describe. In reading her relatively dated article I began to wonder why it is that there is so little mention of this form of reflexivity in the dominant research discourse today. Heshusius contends (and I agree) that there are certainly researchers who live the reflexivity-as-presence mode of consciousness but we simply have not developed a way of communicating about it. Our language is still methodologically based. As May (1982) contends, it seems somehow impossible to explain consciousness-as-content. It is more likely to become known through experience. Certainly I have found it challenging to write about this deep relational presencing in a way that others might come to know and understand it. I eventually came to the conclusion that perhaps the best way to communicate it was not through words but by pointing to examples of it. I came across one such example in an article by Gerber & Harrington (1997). The story told by these authors offers what I see as an example of the power and possibility of reflexivity-as-presencing and how it might complement already existing reflexive practices.

In the article the authors describe the experiences of researchers who listened to Cambodian survivors speak of their experiences before and during the Pol Pot holocaust. The authors describe how the researchers' own meaning constructions and the emotions that arose through those meaning constructions profoundly affected them. In listening to the experiences of the refugees, the researchers wanted to help the refugees feel better. The authors describe how the researchers' reflexive analysis helped them identify what was making the research difficult and causing their anxiety. As I read the article a particular quote from one of the researchers stood out. It describes an experience of a researcher during an interview, and exemplifies the self-abandoned, embodied, relational presence and the heightened feelings and awareness that is accessed through non-action and attentiveness. The following are the researcher's words as he attempts to describe his experience:

> 'I felt like something changed in the room. Like everything else disappeared except for her and me . . . I felt such sadness and heaviness yet I also felt more alive somehow. I felt like there was something more in the room. Words don't do this justice. I know it sounds weird, but it felt like some kind of exchange was happening somewhere between the two of us . . . I felt like we were suspended somewhere in the room . . . and like there was something sacred going on . . . I think that something sacred was happening as she was talking and we were there' (Gerber & Harrington, 1997, p. 60).

This quote depicts how in that relational moment the researcher moved beyond reflexive analysis, beyond the act of stepping back, beyond interpretation, and beyond consciousness with content. In transcending his self-consciousness and his own meaning constructions he accessed consciousness-without-content and ultimately another realm of exchange.

Inquiring into reflexivity has also highlighted how I am living this reflexive presencing in a current research project. A group of colleagues and I are engaged in a study to learn more about the meaning and enactment of 'ethics' in nurses' everyday practice. We have deliberately organised the facilitation of the groups in such a way that one researcher actively observes, records and interprets what is happening in the moment. That is, in an actively reflexive way this researcher's consciousness moves back and forth between self and other in order to observe and interpret. At the same time I, as the other researcher, let go of preoccupations with self, other, observation and interpretation in order to be in a place of complete attention. My attention and awareness are on the life that is welling-up and flowing through us (the nurses and me) as we relationally 'know' the meaningful experience of ethical nursing. This knowing is centred in experience rather than language, cognition, and discourse. And, in a way that is difficult to put into words, this embodied, experiential knowing expands and heightens the depth of understanding and knowledge we are gleaning through our research process.

Reflexive presencing

A final comment about reflexive presencing and consciousness-without-content I wish to make is in relation to the value it has for research participants. It has been my experience that when I am reflexively present in an *inactive* way, the people I am relating with also have the opportunity to 'be' present in that way. This was highlighted during a recent experience I had with a group of women who were talking with me about their experiences of being frontline workers in a shelter for homeless women. As we connected, we moved beyond a cognitive level of discussion and relationally experienced what was similar to the 'sacred' experience the researcher in Gerber & Harrington's (1997) article described above. At the end of our discussion one of the women looked at me and said, 'I have so much appreciated what you had to say. You have the most amazing voice, so inviting and gentle, I could have listened to you all day.' What was so significant about this was that I had actually spoken only a handful of words in the two hours we had been together. This woman had been so reflexively present with myself and the other women and so immersed in her experience and 'knowing' that she had not separated out who had specifically said what. She was aware, however, of the deeper understanding and knowing she had through our time together.

Summary

In conclusion, a quote from Miller Mair (1989) highlights the necessity of paying close attention to how we approach any inquiry and how we live and employ the reflexive process. He states:

> 'Ignoring is an integral part of any knowing, since we have to turn away from what we cannot bear or fear to undertake. We are likely to come to recognize that our ways of ignoring have been developed to an even greater extent than our still timid ways of involving ourselves in the dangerous seas of knowing' (Mair, 1989, p. 7).

It has seemed to me that reflexivity-as-presence might enhance our involvement in deeper and wider realms of knowing. However, it requires that we be willing to move beyond the knowledge and strategies we have developed that help us manage ourselves and oversee the research process. It requires that we at times move beyond managed subjectivity into the fearful sea of self-abandonment, non-action and non-interpreting. It requires something similar to John Caputo's (1987) metaphor of swimming in the abyss:

'... the way one learns to float only by surrendering every attempt to swim and by remaining perfectly still. That takes practice and a bit of courage; it is simple but hard' (1987, p. 224).

References

Caputo, J.D. (1987) *Radical Hermeneutics: Repetition, Deconstruction, and the Hermeneutic Project*. Indiana University Press, Bloomington, Indiana.

Csikszentmihalyi, M. (1993) *The Evolving Self*. HarperCollins Publishers, New York.

Dahlberg, K. & Halling, S. (2000) 'Phenomenological research as the embodiment of openness: swimming upstream in a technological culture'. Paper presented at the *International Human Science Research Conference*, Long Island, New York.

Davies, B. (1993) *Shards of Glass. Children Reading and Writing Beyond Gendered Identities*. Southwood, Sydney, Aus.

Finlay, L. (2002) Negotiating the swamp: the opportunity and challenge of reflexivity in research practice. *Qualitative Research*, **2**(2), 209–30.

Gerber, L. & Harrington, D. (1997) Responsibility and survivor testimony. *The Humanistic Psychologist*, **25**(1), 45–63.

Greene, M. (1995) *Releasing the Imagination. Essays on Education, the Arts, and Social Change*. Jossey-Bass Publishers, San Francisco.

Heshusius, L. (1994) Freeing ourselves from objectivity: managing subjectivity or turning toward a participatory mode of consciousness? *Educational Researcher*, **23**(3), 15–22.

Mair, M. (1989) *Between Psychology and Psychotherapy: A Poetics of Experience*. Routledge, London.

May, G. (1982) *Will and Spirit: A Contemplative Psychology*. Harper & Row, San Francisco, CA.

McNamee, S. (1996) Therapy and identity construction in a postmodern world. In *Constructing the Self in a Mediated World* (Grodin, D. & Lindlof, T.L., eds). Sage Publications, Thousand Oaks, CA.

McNamee, S. & Gergen, K.J. (1999) *Relational Responsibility for a Sustainable Dialogue*. Sage Publications, Thousand Oaks, CA.

Paterson, J. G. & Zderad, L.T. (1976) *Humanistic Nursing*. John Wiley & Sons, New York.

Rorty, R. (1989) *Contingency, Irony, and Solidarity*. Cambridge University Press, Cambridge.

Stanley, L. & Wise, S. (1983) Back into the personal or: our attempt to construct feminist research. In *Theories of Women's Studies* (Bowles, G. & Klein, R., eds). Routledge & Kegan Paul, London.

Varela, F. J., Thompson, E. & Rosch, E. (1993) *The Embodied Mind: Cognitive Science and Human Experience*. The MIT Press, Cambridge, MA.

Weil, S. (1992) *Gravity and Grace*. Routledge, London.

PART III

Reflexivity Within Relationships

Qualitative research involving other people is, rather obviously, a human encounter – and researchers are also human beings! This means that qualitative research scenarios, typically individual or group interviews, are also social interactions, and therefore that understanding the research situation and topic is not pre-given, but *negotiated*. Both researcher and participant will begin with certain (different?) expectations pertaining to the research process, which may or may not be acknowledged, and effort will be expended by both parties to establish a working alliance. Interview questions may not generate the kind of response anticipated or desired by the researcher while the participant might be puzzled or uncertain about the direction in which the interview is going. As researchers, we will find ourselves identifying more with some participants than others, interrupting more, offering personal anecdotes as well as interview questions, and so on. Because of this variability between relatively unique research encounters, researchers need to be aware of, and monitor the effects of, our (inter-)subjective reactions and interventions regarding research participants. In short, reflexivity invites us to reflect on the interactions and relationships worked up in the research setting, and to include such reflections as data in their own right.

In Part III, contributors take seriously their participation in research situations, and offer useful examples of how to manage the issues which this raises. In Chapter 8, Finlay manages both a philosophical and practical exploration as she examines something of the shared intersubjective space between her participants and herself. Drawing upon her research of the therapist's life world, she describes her method of 'hermeneutic reflection', which is artfully conveyed through the metaphor of reflections in the looking glass.

Chapter 9 by Georgaca deploys discourse analysis in order to scrutinise how interview data relating to a 'psychotic' experience is co-constructed by both researcher and participant. Unlike much qualitative analysis, here both the interviewee and the interviewer's conversational turns are subjected to the same rigorous analysis, with a focus mainly on those rhetorical techniques, conversational moves, and discourses invoked. The value of this form of analysis lies in demystifying the role of the interviewer and, in this case, questioning the facile pathologisation of those deemed 'mentally ill'.

Chapter 10 by Nicolson refers to health-related research informed by symbolic interactionism and phenomenology to explore the interaction between inter-viewee and interviewer at different stages in the research process. Using rich data from projects on post-natal depression and stress at work, she clearly documents how the understandings of the topic are the product of meanings shared by both research participants (i.e. interviewer and interviewee). Further, the proactive role of the researcher in facilitating deeper reflection on the part of the participant is underscored. Chapter 11 by Gough also considers interview data but from a broadly psychoanalytic viewpoint. Here, the focus is mainly on the interventions made by the researcher within the research situation – group interviews with male students about 'masculinities'. A 'reflexive voice', which speaks from a suspicious psychoanalytic register, is introduced as a way of interrogating researcher involvement, and a rather disconcerting image of the male researcher as anxious and defensive (in typically 'masculine' ways) is articulated.

CHAPTER 8

Through the looking glass: intersubjectivity and hermeneutic reflection

Linda Finlay

Positioning the self: author's story

My PhD research on the life world of the occupational therapist coincided with my move away from being an occupational therapist to becoming a psychologist and academic. My research, involving interviews with twelve therapists and participant observation, employed interpretivist, phenomenological methodology. Of course I, too, was an occupational therapist and as I was exploring their meanings I was also finding my own.

During my research I struggled with issues around the phenomenological methodology I was gradually, somewhat to my surprise, embracing. How to make sense of the complexities of the data collection and analysis process? How was I to incorporate my feminist, social constructionist leanings? How could I reconcile my socially orientated, relativist beliefs with the apparently individualistic, essentialist understandings embedded in such ideas as 'detached consciousness' and 'bracketing'? How could I set aside my own preconceptions and assumptions as a researcher? Wasn't my social background inextricably intertwined with what I was discovering in my research?

With relief I turned to the existential-phenomenological literature which emphasised how we are always embedded in our social world. I was drawn (not without some ambivalence and misgivings) to Heidegger (1962) and his emphasis on the way that we are pre-reflectively engaged with the world. Gadamer's (1989) hermeneutic circle – where our understandings are seen to be continually modified in a dialectic between pre-understandings and what is being revealed – seemed to make sense. Sartre (1969) helped me to explore the multi-levelled nature of consciousness while Merleau-Ponty showed me the importance of prioritising experience: 'The task of radical reflection . . . consists, paradoxically enough, in recovering the unreflective experience of the world.' (1962, p.241).

Thus, I began to embrace a version of reflexive phenomenology that, some years later, I would call 'hermeneutic reflection'.

Introduction

'Self consciousness is real only in so far as it recognizes its echo (and its reflection) in another' (Hegel, quoted by Sartre, 1969, p.237).

My journey 'through the looking glass' began when I understood that I was a participant in my own research. As an occupational therapist researching other occupational therapists, I was exploring their meanings while simultaneously grappling with my own. I was both subject and object. I was, somehow, reflected in my participants while they (or, perhaps, my understanding of them) were part of me.

My research task was to attempt to explicate the life world of occupational therapists. I adopted an existential-phenomenological approach. With this method, the researcher, the world and the researcher's experience of the world are seen to be intertwined and the focus needs to be on identifying that inter-subjective lived experience which resides in the space between subject and object. How was I to do this when such experience is neither visible nor directly accessible? It wasn't enough to simply 'look in the mirror' (though this was important too). The task required something more than reflecting on either object or subject.

Gradually I learned to move back and forth in a kind of iterative dialectic between experience and awareness, immersing myself in multiple layers of meanings. As Hertz (1997, p.viii) puts it: 'To be reflexive is to have an ongoing conversation about the experience while simultaneously living in the moment.' So I began to construct a version of reflexivity which I have called 'hermeneutic reflection'.

This chapter describes how I engaged, reflexively, throughout the research process from my first approach to my participants through to analysing the data. I start with a brief theoretical/philosophical account of reflexivity as hermeneutic reflection. Then, using examples from my reflexive diary,[1] I describe my initial approach to, and the developing relationships with, my participants. I then give illustrations of reflexive data collection and analysis. At the end of each section, I offer a 'meta-reflexive voice' (located in boxes) – a device to show something more of the layers of reflection involved. A conclusion seeks to draw together these threads and to consider the value and limitations of my version of reflexive analysis.

---

[1] These extracts from my reflexive diary are slightly adapted versions of those presented in my thesis (which is the stated reference, where possible, as this is a more public document).

Box 8.1

Can I 'pull off' this multi-layered use of a mirroring analogy to represent reflection and reflexivity? My starting assumption is that it is through mirroring, when we see ourselves in the reactions of others, that our self-concept and self-understandings arise – Cooley's 'looking glass self'. I apply this in my research to both my participants and myself as we 'reflect back' to each other and 'reflect on' our lived experience. Drawn into self-scrutiny (from catching glimpses of ourselves in the mirror or when we see we're the object of another's attention as in Sartre's 'Look') we become self-conscious and self-aware. It is not sufficient to simply assume the reflection is a true likeness, however. We need to set aside the proposition that the imagery fully encompasses the phenomenon. Instead, we need to ask, 'what in the imagery belongs to the phenomenon and what may distort or hide aspects of it?' We need to look beyond and through the reflection towards a greater sense of what may be there . . .

Reflexivity as hermeneutic reflection

Hermeneutic reflection occurs most explicitly within existential-phenomenological approaches (for instance, Merleau-Ponty, 1962; Sartre, 1969) which argue that:

- Actual (pre-reflective) lived experience can never be fully grasped in its immediate manifestation.
- Our presuppositions and prejudices are both our closedness and openness to the world.
- Every perception is already structured by our interpretations – human access to a world prior to interpretation is impossible.
- Our historicity and situatedness 'determines' our understanding.
- Any understanding we gain (e.g. from research) will inevitably inform us simultaneously about the object of study and about our own preoccupations, expectations and cultural traditions.
- Reflection that aims towards self-awareness – be it in researcher or participant – needs to engage in recovering something of our unreflective experience.

To explain these ideas more fully it may help to view the concepts *hermeneutic* and *reflection* separately.

Hermeneutics emerges out of the work of philosophers such as Heidegger (1962), Gadamer (1975, 1976), and Ricoeur (1981) who argue for our embeddedness in the world of language, ideas and social relationships and for the inescapable historicity of all understanding. Heidegger (1962), for instance, argues that each person will perceive the same phenomenon in a different way, each bringing to bear his or her lived experience, specific understandings and historical background. We experience a thing 'as' something – it has already been interpreted. For Heidegger interpretation is not an additional procedure: it constitutes an inevitable and basic structure of our 'being-in-the-world'. The hermeneutic circle in this context can be understood as a cycle of: (1) foreunderstanding, (2) meeting a 'resistance' when interrogating experience and (3) an interpretative revision of the fore-understanding. Gadamer (1975) picks up the theme in his discussion of the reflexive import of the hermeneutic circle. Given that the method of interpretation is to challenge fore-understanding though addressing the 'thing itself' (initially accessed through the fore-understanding) the process intrinsically involves a self-critique and an ongoing revelation of the assumptions – now found to be partial or wrong – built into the fore-understanding.[2]

Applying these ideas to research, existential-phenomenologists argue that as researchers we cannot help but bring our own involvement into the research. All understandings are inevitably based upon our fore-understandings and pre-judgements. These pre-judgements are both our closedness and our openness to the world – they are the basis of our experiencing. The intrinsic role played by us as interpreters when formulating findings must be acknowledged given the way our perceptions are necessarily entangled when accessing experience. While we should still attempt to disentangle our perceptions and understandings from the phenomenon being studied, we also recognise our interpretations and the ongoing revelation of the thing under scrutiny are one of the same.

Reflexivity is thus the *process of continually reflecting upon our interpretations of both our experience and the phenomena being studied so as to move beyond the partiality of our previous understandings and our investment in particular research outcomes*. Put in Gadamerian terms, reflexivity involves a positive evaluation of the researcher's own experience in order to understand something of the fusion of horizons between subject and object (Gadamer, 1975). Our understanding of 'other-ness' arises through a process of making ourselves more transparent. Without examining ourselves we run the risk of letting our unelucidated prejudices dominate our research findings. New understanding emerges from a complex dialectic between knower and known; between the researcher's past pre-understandings and the present research process, between the self-interpreted co-constructions of both participant and researcher. Between and beyond...

Reflection[3] in the phenomenological sense aims 'to effect a more direct contact with experience as lived' (van Manen, 1990, p.78). To better understand the

---

[2] Readers interested in following up the source of this philosophical exploration might want to read Heidegger's *Being and Time*, section 32 (pages 188–95 in the 1962 Macquarrie and Robinson translation) and Gadamer's *Truth and Method*, pages 265–71.

[3] Reflexivity can often be confused with reflection – and, indeed, in much of the literature these terms are used interchangeably. The concepts are perhaps best viewed on a continuum. Reflection can be understood as 'thinking about' something else (an object). The process is a distanced one and takes place after the event. Reflexivity, in contrast, involves a more immediate, continuing, dynamic and subjective *self*-awareness.

connections between reflection and reflexivity, we can turn to the work of Sartre (1969) where he invites us to examine the fascinating, multi-layered nature of our own consciousness. Sartre distinguishes between: (1) Unreflective consciousness (as such, i.e. *pour-soi*) where the self is an active agent – taken up with living in the moment. At this level, our consciousness is outside the scope of our experience or is lost in the experiencing where we are forgetful of our own agency. (2) Reflective consciousness – here the self and experience can become the object of reflection. (3) Self-reflective consciousness – at this most reflexive level, the self becomes the aim of reflection.[4] These definitions take Sartre away from psychodynamic distinctions of conscious versus unconscious. The point made by Sartre is that it is possible to retrieve our attention and re-focus it on a hitherto ignored aspect. The idea that we can self-reflect on our 'prejudices' and about what we are doing and experiencing adds a further dimension.

Merleau-Ponty (1962, 1968) also pursues this idea of 'radical reflection', arguing that self-comprehension consists, paradoxically, in recovering our unreflective experience. Beyond this, he calls our attention to the way existences (beings) are intertwined in 'a dynamic of reciprocity, a mirroring and doubling' (Levin, 1985, p.256). The being who is a 'toucher' is necessarily 'being touched' simultaneously. It is almost as though to understand something means to have related it to ourselves in such a way that we discover in it an answer to our own question.

Box 8.2

In the section above, I'm aiming to present the theoretical rationale underpinning hermeneutic reflection – a legitimate activity. But what else am I doing? I'm exploiting the (rare) opportunity to expound on philosophy that excites me. That I'm also seeking to persuade you about my construction of 'reflexivity as hermeneutic reflection' is not entirely irrelevant. Most of all, am I not engaged in an exercise of academic self-presentation? All too aware that the examples from my research which follow are prosaic and pragmatic, am I not trying to buttress the argument with some heavyweight theoretical references? Here are my intellectual credentials – see, I too can do philosophy! Perhaps this will backfire ending up a failed strategy which turns you, the reader, off. Yet again, maybe this 'open' confession will gain some sympathy and encourage you to read on?

---

[4] The *self* for Sartre is a transcendent. It is not the same as consciousness nor is it 'part of' consciousness. Consciousness has no intrinsic characteristics. When we turn our attention to our-self, the self becomes the object and we are able to describe our 'characteristics' (though this is, actually, in 'bad faith' as the characteristics of the self can still be changed).

If we apply these ideas to our own research we can appreciate how multiple layers of reflection and reflexivity offer possibilities and opportunities for knowledge. None of us – whether researchers or participants – have privileged access to the 'reality' of our lived experience. When we narrate our experience (be it in an interview or when providing a reflexive account) we offer one version – an interpretation – which seems to work for that moment. Like an external observer, we have to reflect on the evidence and recognise the indexicality and non-con-clusive nature of any of our understandings. 'All reflection is situational ... always subject to revision' (McCleary in Merleau-Ponty, 1962, p.xx).

Approaching the research

The early stages of the research process are particularly crucial for phenomen-ologists for we seek to approach the phenomenon to be investigated with 'openness and awe' – the attitude fundamental to this method. Our first task is to attempt to identify, examine and 'bracket out' presuppositions and pre-understandings in order to enter the lived experience of the participant and to attend genuinely and actively to his or her view. As phenomenologists, we seek to immerse ourselves in the here-and-now, to consciously avoid being distracted by externalities.

Yet to what extent can we actually do this? The problem of phenomenological inquiry, van Manen (1990) explains, is that we know too much. Our common-sense 'pre-understandings, our suppositions, assumptions, and the existing bodies of scientific knowledge, predispose us to interpret the nature of the phe-nomenon before we have even come to grips with the significance of the phe-nomenological question' (1990, p.46). Merleau-Ponty acknowledges the difficulties inherent in the task thus: 'The most important lesson which the reduction [i.e. bracketing process] teaches us is the impossibility of a complete reduction' (1962, p.xiv). Others argue that researchers should at least attempt to make their position explicit to better contextualise any understandings. 'We cannot escape our theoretical presuppositions', argues von Eckartsberg (1986, p.98). 'All we can do is try to make our approach as explicit as possible.'

Applying these ideas to my research, my first task was to reflect – *reflexively!* – on my experience of being a researcher-therapist studying other therapists:

> 'What are my investments in the research? How am I to manage the tensions of being both researcher and therapist? The researcher in me wants to probe and challenge the therapists. The therapist in me wants to "save their face". I want them to perform well and say professionally sound things. This came home forcefully in my second interview when my participant admitted to engaging in a practice which was against unit policy. The researcher-me was quietly excited by this disclosure of covert practice; the therapist-me was

sympathetic, concerned and appalled. Mostly I did not want to hear about it and I wanted to tell her to protect herself and not publicly admit such things!' (Finlay, 1998, p.228)

Below are two further extracts from my reflexive diary which show how I examined my experience in an attempt to bracket it and to better understand my participants. At the same time, I was all too aware how my experience and presuppositions also blocked insights.

In the first extract, I unpack some of the implications of being a therapist myself. Early in my research, I needed to work to unravel instances in which I shared understandings with my participants and ones in which we diverged. I had to guard against assuming that we saw the job in the same way. Without doing some reflexive analysis, I could have missed the point that there were differences:

'In some ways, being an insider is a comfortable and easy role to adopt. I am able to dress and behave as "me". My research participants and I are all white, middle-class therapists, concerned about people, engaged in a project of being "nice". We all went through similar professional socialisation. We share the same language and jargon, even the same jokes. I can identify with them, for example, when they speak of their challenging patients or problematic team relationships. Through understanding my own satisfactions, dilemmas and tensions about being an occupational therapist, I can better understand theirs. My previous knowledge gives me insights which outsiders could not have picked up.

… [Yet] if I make such assumptions I am in danger of missing points of difference. This came home forcefully to me when I started my first participant observation in the field. I started with the assumption (based on my mental health experience) that as therapists we have a fair amount of professional autonomy and that team relationships are reasonably egalitarian. It came as quite a surprise to me to find out how hierarchical some practice could be. Jane, for example, found that no less than a quarter of all her referrals were inappropriate; but she still carried on seeing these clients. When I asked why, the answer came back "because the doctor has requested it, it's prescribed, so I must do it". That was the first time I realised how major some of the differences in our professional experience might be' (Finlay, 1998, p.226–27).

In the second extract, I describe my mixed reactions to donning the uniform I was required to wear in hospital as part of my participant observation. Glancing in the mirror I caught sight of myself in uniform. I panicked. My reactions were so powerful and ambivalent I had to take time to record them there and then. I returned to develop these reflexive notes several times over the week. Here is an excerpt:

(1) 'The uniform is quite nice in that it offers me a sense of being an insider; being accepted and legitimate somehow. This particularly hit me when a

doctor entered into a fairly deep personal and professional conversation with Peter and had automatically included me. Clearly the uniform acts as a sort of passport, and I quite like the inclusion.

(2) The negative side of my experience ... is that I dislike the restraints, the anonymity, the lack of individuality. I find myself wanting to have the staff I am working with (particularly Peter) see me in my usual wear and thus how I "normally" am ...

(3) Then there is the feeling of power which I find myself feeling both negative and positive about. People are passing me in the corridor and giving me what I interpret are "respectful nods". This uniform clearly has some power and I am feeling it too. I have always known I feel negative about this kind of thing; but my positive response to the feeling of power comes as a horrible surprise ...

(4) I notice in the changing rooms at the beginning and end of each day how naturally staff wear and take on and off their uniforms in front of each other. It is part of the routine. It has a practical purpose. But I also sense that they too like the identity/status/belonging that it affords them. Also, they care about the cleanliness etc. of the uniform – it is part of how they "present" themselves' (Finlay, 1998, p.236).

Box 8.3

Gazing at myself in the mirror? . . . Is this not plain vanity and narcissism? Am I simply rationalising my self-focus as legitimate 'research'? Do I seek to do my research merely as an excuse – a cover story – which allows me to look at my reflection, with or without uniform. The answer comes back, 'Yes and No'. 'Yes', because I know the very choice of research topic has arisen from my own preoccupations. I have an interest and an investment in the outcomes, a 'passion' even. 'No', because I also have a genuine desire to understand the other's experience – to celebrate what we share and how we differ. I know I have come into the research with my own ideological baggage about what occupational therapy is and should be. I want these understandings to be challenged. I want to see the world differently, to learn. Don't I?

Maybe the lesson here is that Narcissus wasn't reflexive enough. Had he been more *self*-aware as opposed to mesmerised by the reflection of himself as an 'other', perhaps he would not have fallen in love with himself . . .

Developing relationships with participants

The two examples above begin to show the role and value of reflexive analysis in clarifying the impact of the researcher's position and perspective. This analysis needs to be extended to similarly encompass intersubjective dynamics. In particular, researchers need to attend to the evolving relationship between themselves and their participants. In my own research, there were numerous occasions where the interactions and relationship dynamics between my participants and myself clearly influenced the stories that emerged and the depth and quality of the subsequent analysis. Two examples, again taken from my reflexive diary, illustrate this.

(1) 'My interview with Paula felt largely out of my control. She talked a lot and quite quickly, such that I did not feel able to get a word in without being assertive. Yet, I was content to simply listen and let her take the interview where she chose. Much of the information she gave was new to me and I wanted to learn. I also warmed to her and enjoyed her company. She, in turn, blossomed in the face of my evident interest' [extract from Reflexive Diary]

(2) 'Jane was much more reticent and reserved. She did not initiate any disclosures, which in turn made me much more active. I felt pushed to ask more questions and I became (reluctantly) much more directive. In the process I ended up asking what was for me an unusually large number of closed questions. Did I sense a vulnerability in her and, by asking closed questions, was trying to protect her from disclosing too much? Interestingly, Jane, more than any of the other therapists, got me disclosing more to her. She took the initiative to ask me questions, and I obliged, partly in my desire to share something with her in return. I also felt a need to confide in her. From the first moment I felt drawn to her as a therapist and as a beautiful woman. Somehow I wanted a part of her niceness and nurturing – perhaps even be her client? At the same time I could see that her general "niceness", combined with her controlling quality (with her asking me questions) and lack of self-disclosure, were all effective defences in stopping me from pushing or challenging her. Jane and I, together, seemed to be engaged in an exercise to stop me probing too much' (Finlay, 1998, p.240–42).

Box 8.4

It's like seeing simultaneous reflections in multiple mirrors. As I dwell with the transcripts of conversations between participants and myself, the images become blurred and identities converge. The therapist I am interviewing becomes my client. The 'I' who is both researcher and therapist divides and I slide inadvertently into my therapist body. As therapist I feel a familiar sensation in my belly – a stirring of excitement as emotional empathy expands. I experience a sense of 'humble power'. I feel honoured as the participant opens herself, discloses secrets, shares her tears. I know something of the power I have used to 'facilitate' this. Yet, simultaneously, I feel powerless and helpless.

Cont.

Box 8.4   *Cont.*

What can I do in the face of this distress? I am not her therapist. Then, as I witness her strength, wisdom, caring, I am reminded that she is a therapist herself with a capacity and her own ways to cope. Then images converge again and a new relationship comes into focus. Suddenly, I am the client, feeling tears, needing solace, wanting this caring, listening therapist to nurture and reassure me. Then a point of interest captures my professional attention. The axis spins, and I find myself being the researcher. I can stand back now and draw a cloak of power around me once more as I select what to hear, what to report. I decide how to represent my participants and which stories I tell. Will I tell of my own struggle to both hold together and separate my therapist, client and researcher selves? I'm not sure . . .

Collecting data

Wertz (1984) has argued for researchers to reflect vigorously on their data collection process:

> 'The researcher's use of descriptions is not based on a naïve acceptance of verbal data per se. Rather she is forced to reflect rigorously on the particular problems each research project poses ... The same is generally true of the role of the researcher whose presence, for example in observation and interviews, can be responsible for omissions and even fabrications which are mistaken as valid data' (Wertz, 1984, p.39).

These dilemmas confronted me as I interviewed therapists about their experience. Deep and sometimes painful reflection was required before I could begin to unravel the multiple and shifting meanings within my participants' responses. On the positive side, it became clear that insights could emerge from examining one's own ambivalent responses. It is these ambivalent responses that alert the researcher to the need to be reflexive. Two examples from my research stand out:

(1) 'On one occasion I was observing an occupational therapist work with a client who was suffering from the final stages of lung cancer. Although I was supposed to only observe, I found I could not stop myself becoming involved (by asking the patient questions and even intervening at a practical level). When I reflected on my behaviour, I understood it was my active need to be involved – to do something. I also recognised my own sensitivity as an asthmatic, witnessing someone with breathing problems dying of a lung disease. Once I recognised this, I could then see the occupational therapist was experiencing similar identifications with some of her other patients. Previously I had interpreted the therapist as

being involved with fairly superficial, "irrelevant" tasks – now I could see these tasks had a meaning for her: they were as much for her as the patient. By examining my own responses I could better understand hers' (Finlay, 1998, p.454).

(2) '[With one of my participants] I found myself feeling irritated with what I saw as a cold, mechanical approach; one that was inappropriate in a therapist. I found myself being uncharacteristically challenging with him. I pushed him to get an emotional response. Then, towards the end of the interview he opened up and spoke, quite painfully, about how difficult it was to handle certain emotions and how he had to cut himself off from them at work. I then felt guilty for having been so insensitive and forcing such disclosures. Reflecting on this I wondered about the extent to which I set all that up with my initial assumptions. To what extent did he produce behaviours, both the mechanical and emotional, because I was inviting them? ...

Having engaged in reflexive analysis ... [I concluded] that I had probably influenced my informant. In addition, I came to understand that the multiple, contradictory ideologies around in our culture also had a considerable influence and that emotions reflect our ideologies ... For one thing I suspect my informant had internalised the same messages I have about "acceptable" gender behaviour. But I also saw that he would have been exposed to other ideologies; for instance, how as professionals we should be empathetic and emotional, as well as professional and in control of our feelings. My negative reactions probably reflected the society within which the occupational therapist practised and had to struggle. In this way, my reflections (about my own assumptions, society's ideas and my informant's inconsistent presentation) became part of the research data I needed to take note of and analyse' (Finlay, 1998, p.454).

Box 8.5

'I found myself being uncharacteristically challenging.' A classic use of rhetoric! Yet in my defence, it is understandable why I feel the need to distance myself from this negative behaviour. I am ashamed (shame coming from being subjected to Sartre's judging, objectifying 'Look'?) of my blatant manipulations and use of power in the way I have marshalled my therapist skills. What gives me this right? Is my way out simply to assert the participant was responsible for himself? I am reminded how difficult it can be for the researcher to reveal personal fragility and methodological inadequacy. And, then, in making this fresh rhetorical move to reveal my failings am I not just trying to justify and excuse them? Am I not inoculating myself against likely protests that I am offering a 'partial' (in both senses of the word) account and showing that I can, at least, recognise and 'atone' for (some of) my mistakes?

Data analysis

Carrying out reflexive data analysis is always problematic. Such understanding is difficult to unfold – our experience is invariably complex, ambiguous, ambivalent. Much commitment, care, time, and skill go into reflexive analysis, and to do it well takes practice. Immersing oneself in one's data can prove a painful business. Personal insights, when they arise, can be uncomfortable. However, researchers committed to the reflexive project need to be prepared for these eventualities and to probe their more disagreeable reactions. As instruments of our own research, we need to engage in such analysis, however burdensome this may be (Kleinman, 1991).

Preoccupations with one's own emotions and experiences can pull research in unfortunate and undesirable directions. For one thing it can unduly privilege the researcher's voice at the expense of the participants'. As researchers, we need to strike some balance between self-awareness and undue navel gazing. The following excerpt indicates how self-experience can be exploited while the researcher attempts to maintain the primary focus on the participant:

> 'I found myself feeling angry with a therapist participant. My anger was stopping me from listening and empathising and I needed to examine what was happening. I was feeling angry on behalf of a patient who needed to stay longer in hospital to complete a range of crucial assessments, but the therapist was unable to challenge the doctors who were intent on discharging the patient. On reflection, I interpreted that my anger mirrored the therapist's anger at herself. She regularly put herself down for not communicating more assertively with doctors. On delving deeper, I located what appeared to be the *real* source of both our angers: the hierarchical system investing the doctor with such power. This then became a key theme in my generic analysis of the life world of occupational therapists. By reflecting on our shared emotional responses, I was led to locate the context that prompted those responses and to recognise its importance in shaping how therapists experience their work' (Finlay, 1998, pp.454–5).

One of the most powerful moments in my data analysis occurred when I was analysing an excerpt from my interview with a mental health therapist who had been threatened by some male patients with a violent sexual history. She described, at some length, her sense of apprehension that one predatory patient would eventually 'get her'. Here is an extract from the interview:

> *Jenny:* 'He's ... extremely creepy. He will come up, want to touch you ... He's a bit predatory in that he will follow you down corridors ... He preyed across the gym ... crept up behind me ... "They [colleagues] can't watch all of you all the time ... I'll get you." ... He even does things like, there's a large observation window, and even if he can't physically get to you, he'll stand

there and rub his groin and drool ... He'll crawl across the floor to get you' [Interview 8, pp.10–11].

In my analysis of this interview, I found myself reading and re-reading the transcript with a growing sense of foreboding. I started to imagine how I would feel in Jenny's shoes, stalked by this predator:

'Suddenly, the world begins to look different. Everything closes round me and somehow grows darker. I can hear the hollow beating of my heart. I think about the unit Jenny works in, seeing it now in terms of the spaces that are safe versus dangerous. She has to walk down public corridors all the time with full awareness she is not "safe". I feel her fear, that sense of menace where time is no defence. I experience her loathing, her disgust. The image of a man drooling and clawing at the window won't go away. It feels real, like that has happened to me. It is if I have become Jenny' [Extract from Reflexive Diary].

Box 8.6

This is the moment I wait for in my phenomenological analysis: the moment where I am so immersed in the data and intertwined with my participant I can no longer separate the pieces. As Merleau-Ponty has expressed it: 'to the extent that I understand, I no longer know who is speaking and who is listening' (1964, p.97). Words, images, sensations, emotions all converge – all feel so 'loud' somehow. The messages for my analysis become clear! ... Then, the doubts and questions begin to creep in once more. Just who am I talking about? To what extent might I be imagining Jenny's reaction, imposing my own experience in a desperate attempt to empathise? Where is the dividing line between my own experience and that of the creative writer capable of getting 'inside' a character? Might this all just be an excuse to 'play' with my own emotions through the fairy tales I am weaving? Is this study of mine simply a reflection of my personal, as opposed to shared, emotional responses? Can it be anything else?

Summary

This chapter has explored some of the different ways I have used hermeneutic reflection. Examples have illustrated how I examined my experience in order to attempt to bracket it, as well as to better understand my participants and the impact of our relationship. I have tried to demonstrate how reflexivity can be exploited in research to promote insight and how it might aid understanding lived experience. The examples given (from examining intersubjective responses to employing the meta-reflexive voice) have sought to show some of the different layers of analysis involved.

Positioning myself and my perspective explicitly has helped me to evaluate my research while also opening up my research decisions and findings to public scrutiny. I would have to stop short of claiming that reflexivity can *ensure* the trustworthiness and integrity of research. However, I would defend its role in forcing me to stay mindfully engaged. Doing reflexive analysis has also sharpened my capacity for self-criticism, alerting me to the possibility that reflexivity can be used as a strategy for claiming authority. Furthermore, I have learnt that no single account can be anything other than 'partial', emergent and tentative. In the last analysis, qualitative research seeks to capture and reveal the multiple, ambiguous, slippery meanings and images within our social world. Reflexive analysis allows something of these multiple images to be reflected. In using 'a mirror of moving shadows' (McCleary quoted in Merleau-Ponty, 1962, p.xviii), however, we must never mistake our reflections for reality.

Yet, as reflexivity continually challenges our practices and understandings, a truth is revealed: 'Since the seer is caught up in what he sees, it is still himself he sees. There is a fundamental narcissism of all vision' (Merleau-Ponty, 1968, p.138). Hermeneutic revelation of the phenomenon and reflexive uncovering of the self are one.

Acknowledgement

My special thanks go to Professor Peter Ashworth, Sheffield Hallam University, for his wise guidance in shaping my understandings of both phenomenology and reflexivity.

References

Finlay, L. (1998) *The Life World of the Occupational Therapist: Meaning and Motive in an Uncertain World*. PhD thesis, The Open University.

Gadamer, H.-G. (1975) *Truth and Method*. Seabury Press, New York.

Gadamer, H.-G. (1976) *Philosophical Hermeneutics* (translated and edited by D.E. Linge). University of California Press, Berkeley.

Heidegger, M. (1962) *Being and Time*. Harper and Row, New York.

Hertz, R. (1997) Introduction: reflexivity and voice. In *Reflexivity and Voice* (Hertz, R., ed.). Sage Publications, Thousand Oaks, CA.

Kleinman, S. (1991) Field-workers' feelings: what we feel, who we are, how we analyze. In *Experiencing Fieldwork: An Inside View of Qualitative Research* (Shaffier, W.B. & Stebbins, R.A., eds). Sage Publications, Newbury Park, CA.

Levin, D.M. (1985) *The Body's Recollection of Being: Phenomenological Psychology and the Deconstruction of Nihilism*. Routledge & Kegan Paul, London.

Merleau-Ponty, M. (1962) *Phenomenology of Perception*. Routledge & Kegan Paul, London.

Merleau-Ponty, M. (1964) *Signs*. Northwestern University Press, Evanston.

Merleau-Ponty, M. (1968) *The Visible and the Invisible*. Northwestern University Press, Evanston.

Ricoeur, P. (1981) *Hermeneutics and the Human Sciences*. Cambridge University Press, New York.

Sartre, J.-P. (1969) *Being and Nothingness*. Routledge, London.

van Manen, M. (1990) *Researching Lived Experience: Human Science for an Action Sensitive Pedagogy*. State University of New York Press, New York.

von Eckartsberg, R. (1986) *Life-World Experience: Existential-Phenomenological Research Approaches in Psychology*. University Press of America, Washington DC.

Wertz, F.J. (1984) Procedures in phenomenological research and the question of validity. In *Exploring the Lived World: Explorations in Phenomenological Psychology* (Aanstoos, C.M., ed.) West Georgia College Studies in the Social Sciences, Vol. 23. West Georgia College, Carrollton.

CHAPTER 9

Analysing the interviewer: the joint construction of accounts of psychotic experience

Eugenie Georgaca

Positioning the self: author's story

For the past 15 years I have been interested in non-pathologising and empowering ways of understanding and dealing with human distress. This interest has led me to research 'psychotic speech', the speech disturbances of individuals diagnosed as psychotic. While reviewing the literature, I was struck by the way mainstream psychiatric research perpetuates the notion that psychotic speech is pathological. This is done by systematically ignoring the context within which speech is produced. For example, patients' speech is elicited through research interviews. Yet their speech is taken out of context and analysed as a symptom of some underlying pathology, not as a response to a particular interactional situation. As a result, 'psychotic speech' appears incoherent.

These findings made me aware that different research practices were needed, with reflexivity as their key element. I could only hope to understand the speech of my interviewees if I took into account the way I designed my research and interacted with them, analysing it as something produced in the context of a research project and as a response to my interventions. This, of course, changed the nature of my research questions. 'Incoherent' talk was analysed in terms of the functions it served in the interview. 'Delusional' talk was analysed in terms of how claims to what is happening to the person are negotiated between us. Through treating the participants in the study as subjects rather than objects and through investigating what sense their speech might make in the interactional context, a different picture of psychotic speech emerged.

In the past few years, as a trainee Lacanian psychotherapist, my research interests have shifted to analysing the process of psychotherapy, with emphasis on the changes in the clients' subjectivity through the interaction with the therapist. Reflexivity, both in terms of my role as a researcher and of the theoretical and methodological choices I make, is also a key aspect of this research project.

Introduction

Reflexivity is a widely used – and misused – concept in discourse analytic research. In this chapter, I will focus on the use of reflexive principles in the process of analysing and presenting interview material. Through the analysis of extracts from an interview I conducted, I will highlight the constitutive role of the interviewer in the production of research 'data' and argue for the usefulness of subjecting the interviewer's interventions to the same analysis as that of the interviewees. My aim is to show that a reflexive discourse analysis can interrogate how knowledge is discursively constructed both in terms of the interactional production of the interview material and in terms of the production of professional knowledge about mental illness.

I will first discuss the way in which different aspects of reflexivity have informed the analysis of the interview and then present the extracts. The interview presented here was part of a project on 'psychotic' discourse, a critique of mainstream psychiatric theory and research on mental illness drawing upon social constructionism and discourse analysis (Georgaca, 1996). This critical stance is retained throughout the analysis and the last section of the chapter examines the contribution of reflexivity to empowering research on mental illness.

Defining reflexivity

Burr (1995) summarised two main ways in which the notion of reflexivity has been used in discourse research. The first refers to the implications of the view of *speech as action*. Reflexive research acknowledges that participants' talk both describes phenomena and constitutes them through describing them. The second notion of reflexivity refers to the acknowledgement that since all knowledge is *discursively produced* then discourse research should be subjected to the same scrutiny concerning its knowledge-producing assumptions and practices. Discourse researchers need to be attentive to the ways in which their own practices in research design, participation and analysis constitute a particular kind of knowledge (Burman, 1992). At a more global level, the researcher needs to be aware of the historical contingency of discourse research and the necessity to reflexively examine its role within wider scientific research (Parker, 1994). I will examine the way each of these aspects informs my research in turn, with particular reference to the analysis presented in the following sections.

Descriptions and constructions

For discourse theorists, science is not a neutral and objective strategy for discovering what is in the internal world of individuals or the external world of objects; rather, it is a highly regulated system of social practices which constitute and reproduce objects of knowledge (Mulkay & Gilbert, 1985; Myers, 1985). This is because the scientific tools one uses are already products of, and productive of, the social world. In addition, scientists approach the social world already carrying with them assumptions which partake of the same social world they attempt to study. Moreover, texts and discourses construct positions from which they can be read, analysed and understood (Barthes, 1987]; Wetherell, 1998). Despite the attempt to attain an objective position, *the researcher is always caught up in the subject positions constructed by the text*. This especially applies when the researcher is also a participant in the production of the text, in the case of this research as both the interviewer and the analyst.

The acknowledgement that researchers approach their object of study both as representatives of the scientific institution and as social actors subjectively implicated in the production of texts provides a constant tension in the process of analysing an interview (see the debate between Leudar & Antaki, 1996a, b and Potter, 1996b). In my capacity as an interviewer and a discourse analyst, I drew upon culturally available expectations about the ways in which conversations function and about the kinds of claims that can be made and the strategies through which they can be negotiated. As a researcher analysing the interview, I was called upon to employ scientifically refined methods to understand the interactional dynamics. The analysis of the material was a dialectical process taking place between my common-sense understanding of the conversational processes, and a careful, detailed and technical reading of the formal properties of the text. Throughout this process I did not treat my common-sense understanding of the text as naïve or less valid than a 'scientific' and technical reading of it. Rather, I took them to be two poles of a tension, and I constantly used one to test, understand and enhance the other.

Analysing the interviewer

One aspect of reflexive practice is that the discourse researcher should be attentive to the ways in which their own practices in research design, participation and analysis constitute a particular kind of knowledge. Here I will deal with only one aspect of this: the constitutive role of the researcher as interviewer. The interviewer is not passive and does not simply pose questions in order to elicit interviewees' responses. The interviewer's questions evoke specific types of responses and produce particular types of positions for both the interviewer and the interviewee. Moreover, the interviewer approaches the interviewees' speech as a social actor, carrying cultural assumptions about how talk develops and what counts as appropriate rules for conversation, and drawing upon culturally available discourses about the nature of external reality, society and subjectivity. The interviewer's role is that of a socially competent participant, whose discursive practices are subject to the same types of laws and regulations as any other speaker's (Banister *et al.*, 1994).

While these dynamics are readily acknowledged in discourse literature, the interviewer's role is usually ignored in the presentation of interview material, where the interviewer's interventions are often either left out or are not analysed (Leudar & Antaki, 1996a). In this study, my interventions are subjected to the *same analysis* as the interviewee's talk. The linguistic and rhetorical techniques I use, the conversational moves I make, the discourses I draw upon and the positions I make available for myself and the interviewee, are extensively analysed. The analysis of my role in the interview process becomes even more pertinent since my position as a researcher and/or a representative of the psychiatric staff creates an asymmetrical situation in which my interventions have more power in defining the situation and driving the conversational dynamic than the interviewee's. My double position as a social actor and as a researcher and/or psychiatric staff provides a constant tension both in the interview dynamic itself and in the analysis of my active role in constituting the conversation.

Presenting the analysis

The interview with the person I will call July took place on the second day of her admission in an acute psychiatric ward. July is a black African woman in her late twenties. At the beginning of the interview, July claims that the reason she was voluntarily admitted is that one day she realised that people knew about her life and said bad things about her, which overwhelmed and distressed her. These claims can be clearly classified according to psychiatric criteria (APA, 1994) as 'persecutory delusions'. After my questioning regarding the nature of that experience, July arrives at the claim made in the first extract (Box 9.1), which is diagnosable as 'auditory hallucination', a central feature of schizophrenia.

My question at the beginning of the extract is a demand for information about

---

Box 9.1   Extract 1 – Establishing the 'facts'

Interviewer: Hmm so . . . did something happen that made that specific day so bad?
July: Well . . . I felt a bit more . . . nothing happened, it's just that one day it's like just, things came to my mind, and . . . I was just, I was listening and somebody was reporting to me . . . so . . . so I sat er, I couldn't go out because I didn't have the courage to go out.
I: Yeah . . .
I: Was it the feeling that it was somebody else or was it like yourself reporting to you?
J: Oh, I don't know . . . [laughter].
I: [laughter].

the cause of July's distress. July's initial reaction ('I felt a bit more (...) nothing happened') describes the event as a feeling. In her subsequent formulation, however, she establishes the experience of perception ('I was listening') and the existence of an external force or entity which is the cause of that perception ('things came to my mind', 'somebody was reporting to me'). The passage fluctuates between describing listening as a pure subjective experience and establishing the existence of an external entity to which this experience relates. This fluctuation expresses problems inherent in the common-sense understanding of perception. The subjective experience of perception cannot be negotiated, since it belongs to the domain of the experience of one's internal state (Shotter, 1981). Perception is also, however, the product of one's observation of external reality. In cases where no observable stimulus can be established, the status of perception as a reflection of the external world is brought into question and has to be accounted for in terms of the perceiver dreaming, imagining it or being mentally ill (Pollner, 1987).

My formulation of July's claims (Heritage & Watson, 1979) articulates exactly this dilemma. I take for granted her subjective experience, which I classify, nevertheless, not as perception but as feeling, which is a typical way of dealing with claims whose status is considered to be problematic (Coulter, 1975), and then I question the source of this experience. Following the two poles of the dilemma, I formulate two possibilities for the source of July's experience: it could either be an external entity ('somebody else') or her internal processes ('yourself reporting to you'). July's reaction and the laughter that follows establishes both her recognition of the terms of the dilemma I am posing and her problems in either discarding it through the use of another framework or definitely locating herself in either of these poles. The first pole would drive her to a situation of claiming the existence of something which is unusual and which she cannot substantiate. The implication would be that her position as a competent social actor would be undermined. The second pole implies that she misperceives reality because of some internal defect. Accepting this would, therefore, undermine her rationality and integrity as well as her credentials as a responsible bearer of claims on her experience and on reality.

In terms of the reflexive analysis of this extract, it is quite clear that both July and myself present ourselves as competent social actors, sharing assumptions about the nature of perception and internal experience. Moreover, it is me, as the interviewer, who articulates the difficult dilemma that will be negotiated in the rest of the interview. In the next extracts, I examine how the two poles are negotiated using different discourses. These demonstrate how the location of July's distress to having heard a voice allows her to gradually distance herself from it and assume an independent position away from its influence.

At the beginning of the extract in Box 9.2, I ask July to provide the account her friends have given about her situation. Enquiring about possible alternative accounts constitutes a challenge to the consensual character of July's account.

Box 9.2 Extract 2 – Negotiating reality and subjectivity through medical discourse

Interviewer: What do your friends say about it?

July: They say, I told one of my friends and she said it's part of the illness.

I: Mm hmm.

I: Do you believe that?

J: I don't really, to be honest, but I have to believe it [laughter] I have no choice, I mean what can I do?

I: [laughter].

J: [laughter].

I: Yeah, yeah . . . that's right . . . yeah, because you, you believe that all these are really happening , , , don't you?

J: [sigh].

I: Yeah, I know . . . I'm putting difficult questions.

J: [laughter].

I: [laughter] . . . I know, sorry [laughter].

Consensus is an issue appealed to by speakers for the establishment of the veracity of their claims, and the lack of it is appealed to by co-participants to question claims (Edwards & Potter, 1992). In this case, my question about consensus is an indirect statement of my reservations concerning the validity of July's statements. July provides her friends' account by evoking medical discourse. My request that she positions herself in relation to this account clearly puts her in a difficult position. Accepting that she is ill implies disclaiming both the factuality of her experience and her personal integrity. Her response is a strategic move of neither accepting nor disclaiming it. My response to her diplomatic move is constructed as a formulation of the gist of her previous argument and framed as a contrast between July being ill and 'all this really happening'. In other words I impose a frame according to which July's perception of the voice can be explained by either a real external stimulus or by her being ill. The terms in which the dilemma is constructed by me leave July in an impossible situation. The sigh and laughter that follows are signs of the difficulty July has in assuming either of these positions, and the issue is given up after my apologies.

The appeal to medical discourse is well-grounded in the context of the interview. The positions available to participants within the medical framework are severely restricted to the polarity between that of the professional, researcher or doctor, and that of the patient. In this extract, my demand that July positions herself in relation to medical discourse, is also a demand on her to assume the position of the patient, a position which July is explicitly reluctant to assume. Later in the interview, I am implicitly adopting the position of a researcher or doctor within a medical framework by constructing myself as an independent observer of July's situation and authorising myself to offer explanations for her condition, by appealing to her religious convictions and the fact the she lives in a foreign country.

In this extract (as in Box 9.1) both July and myself share common understandings about conversational rules as well as about the implications of evoking the category of mental illness. And again, it is I who, through creating a polarity between July being mentally ill and 'all this really happening', forces July to a difficult position and I undermine her claims. The positions of myself as a 'researcher' and 'interviewer' – the dominant party in the exchange – and July as an 'interviewee' and 'psychiatric patient', is not just an objective feature of the interview; it is rather actively constructed during the interview, and especially through my interventions. Up to this point in the interview the subjective reality of July's experience has been constructed as a non-negotiable fact, and the source of this experience has been negotiated through this two-pole construction. The analysis of the following extracts will focus on the construction of the content of the voice's statements and the negotiation of July's position towards it.

My first question in Box 9.3 refers to the issue of sin and guilt that July has been discussing in previous parts of the interview. My request that she objectively

---

Box 9.3   Extract 3 – Negotiating positions towards the voice

Interviewer: Do you feel that your life was kind of exceptionally . . . bad, you've done more bad things than anybody else?

July: Yeah, yeah, yeah, I mean, yeah, I didn't think that thing, but, that, that night a couple of days ago, when I heard this voice that said . . . it's because of me that my own country is starving . . . my own country is starving and it's because of me . . . because I was, I don't really know, I don't know what I did, it did say what I did, but it's related to my sin.

I: Mm hmm.

J: What I did, and the country has got no end of problems but it's related to my sin.

I: Do you believe that?

J: I don't believe that . . . I just, I was, I was not in any position towards that, I mean . . . how can I, I, I don't know, I couldn't believe, I mean, I said I, I, was I, was I somebody else before and now another person? [laughter] You know.

I: [laughter].

J: I don't know.

I: Is it real things that you did, that you're . . . accused about?

J: Yeah, some of, yeah, some of them, yes, in fact, like I, I didn't care, I didn't care about my family and, I mean, I betrayed my family.

I: Mm hmm.

J: And that's really but I mean it's . . . er, yeah, that's true.

I: Yeah.

J: That's true, but . . . but when it comes to a country level or something, you know?

judges her actions in comparison to the actions of other people is based on the assumption that the feeling of guilt should be distinguished from the 'objective' judgement of the person's 'real' actions. July's answer fluctuates between her dismissal of the view that she has sinned more than others and the voice's claims that the starvation of her country is the result of her sin. The content of the voice's claims is for the first time introduced here. The voice's claims are implicitly offered as a strong counter-argument to July's judgement, as something that should be taken as a valid claim. Her own subjective judgement is partly contrasted to and partly merged with the all-encompassing character of the voice. July's speaker status is problematic, as she appears to animate the voice's claims without taking responsibility for her own claims (Goffman, 1981).

Again, as with the rest of the contents of subjective experience, the content of the voice's claims is taken for granted by both. My subsequent question, however, opens up another possible subjective position for July. It constructs 'her' as different from 'the voice' and asks her to assume a position which is different from it, the position of the 'author' and the 'principal' of her own words, as opposed to an 'animator' of the voice's claims (Goffman, 1981). Her response expresses her being taken aback and her ambivalence about whether to take up that position. Her initial rejection of the voice's claims ('I don't believe that') is subverted by her drawing back to an inability to assume a separate position ('I just, I was, I was not in any position towards that'), followed by hesitations and uncertainty ('how can I, I, I don't know, I couldn't believe, I mean') and ends up with the assumption of an attitude towards the voice and the use of an interpretative framework to disclaim the voice's statements.

My next question appeals to 'reality' and asks July to define which of the accusations the voice has proffered are 'real'. In the framework I evoke the assessment of what the voice accuses her of has to be based on the observation of reality and the objective investigation of her actions. July complies with this by enumerating her 'real' wrong-doings and by implication distinguishing between her 'real' sins and the 'non-real' parts of the voice's accusations. Formulated in the form of a question, she ends up assuming the requested position and challenging the voice.

In this extract, a significant move was accomplished. July gradually moved from merging with the voice to distancing herself from it and questioning the validity of the voice's claims. Through the analysis of the extract I showed how this was done interactionally, through my interventions which cut across July's frame and created a different subject position for her, which she reluctantly but gradually assumed. In the next extract in Box 9.4, this process will be completed by July distancing herself both from the voice and from my own positioning of her through a framework she introduces, namely that of religious discourse.

My first question in this extract is a challenge to July's feeling distressed as a result of the voice's claims, through a contrast between her not believing everything the voice says and her feeling bad about it. The assumption behind my statement is

---

Box 9.4 Extract 4 – Distancing herself

Interviewer: I don't understand, because if you don't, if you don't believe . . . in everything that the voice says . . . I mean, why do, why do you feel so bad about it?
July: I mean, I believe I, I, I believe, I mean, I believe I mu-, I must have made mistakes, and . . . I believe in this, I've gone too far . . . 'cos, I mean, if you see things in religious, in religious terms and they are far advanced, far away from er, er whatever, so I feel bad about it, I know people do bad things, I mean, I know people who are like me.
I: Mm hmm.
J: They could be worse than me but.
I: Hmm.
J: It, it depends how you take it, and personally I find myself guilty.
I: Hmm.
J: But er I think I do mistakes every time . . . sometimes intentionally, sometimes without knowing, you know, it just happens.
I: Yeah.
J: I do believe that, you know, it's always since I was hearing the voices . . . that it always there, you know, that, that, that it had nothing to do with me.
I: What?
J: It has nothing to do with me, er.
I: What do you mean?
I: Are you saying that the voice has nothing to do with you?
J: No, some of the sayings that the voice tells me have nothing to do with me.
I: Yeah . . . hmm.

---

that feelings are formed through and are consequences of judgements. This is part of the intellectualist tradition of the primacy of cognitive functions and the derivative character of affect which is characteristic of Western culture (Gaines, 1992). July's response is initially characterised by hesitations acknowledging both the need and her inability to resolve the inconsistency. Her way out of this is achieved through the appeal to religious discourse. She justifies her feelings of guilt not in terms of observing reality and comparing her sins to others', as she did after my suggestion in the previous extract, but in terms of a judgement of herself based on religious principles. While in the previous extracts July is gradually assuming a position which is independent from the voice, she is still located within the framework of 'rationality', consistency, independence and objective judgement – a position which I had imposed on her during the interview. In this extract, she manages the assumption of a separate position, with respect to both the voice and the position I constructed for her, through the appeal to religious discourse as an alternative interpretative framework. Here, the appeal to religion is shifted from a factor contributing to her illness to a framework that justifies her experience and positions her as an independent thinking individual.

Psychiatric criteria and the discursive construction of facts

A key thread of our interview is a construction and negotiation of 'the facts' that led July to hospital admission. Different versions of 'what actually happened' are produced in the course of the interview. The shifting of the facts is not a gradual uncovering of the 'truth' of what happened – the 'reality' of July's experience. The reality of July's experience is something *interactionally constructed* during the interview. However, it is constructed *as if* it were an unravelling of the real facts. Moreover, the shifts in the way that reality is constructed serve interactional and rhetorical aims (Potter, 1996a). At the beginning of the interview, July appears overwhelmed by an experience which causes her distress and whose type and content she is unable to define. Introducing the fact of July having heard a voice allows her to establish an experience of a definable type (Extract 1) and content (Extract 3). From then on, the content of the voice's claims is taken for granted and the subject of negotiation becomes July's attitude towards the voice's claims. This is initially pursued through an appeal to her 'real' sins and later through an appeal to religious discourse (Extract 4). This opens the possibility for July to gradually assume a position towards that experience and become the 'author' of her own words (Extracts 3 and 4). July's position, therefore, shifts from the passive position of being subjected to an experience she can neither define nor control, to assuming an active position of differentiating herself from, and being critical of, that experience.

The negotiation of 'what happened' throughout the interview follows typical conversational rules and common-sense assumptions. Both July and myself assume that 'what happened' is a fact that has to be unravelled; we follow assumptions about the nature of external reality and subjective experiences. In doing so, we both conduct ourselves as competent social actors. Although constructed as an independent pursuit of truth, our negotiations are formed through a specific interpretative framework: that of equating rationality with common-sense reasoning procedures. In the last extract, July differentiates herself from this framework through the use of an alternative framework – that of religious discourse. In this way she preserves her credentials as a competent social actor, while distancing herself from the specific image of rationality that I had imposed on her.

The negotiation of facts and positions also takes place with reference to the discourses of the psychiatric institution. The negotiation of positions within psychiatric discourse is inextricably linked to the status of participants and their power to define reality (Georgaca, in press). In the interview this takes two forms. Firstly, there is an explicit negotiation of the positions available within psychiatric discourse. I position myself as a researcher or doctor who has the right to examine July's experience (Extracts 1 and 2). I also both explicitly (Extract 2) and implicitly (Extract 1) position her as a psychiatric patient, which July is forced to reluctantly assume (Extract 2). Secondly, the negotiation of positions takes place more indirectly, through the equation of normality with rationality. I repeatedly question July on the basis of her rationality or request that she assumes a rational position towards her claims (Extracts 1, 3 and 4). July assumes that position and responds from within it. It is only in the last extract that July escapes those positions and assumes an independent stance for evaluating her experience through the adoption of religious discourse as an alternative empowering framework.

The analysis of extracts from this interview constitutes a challenge to the psychiatric definition of delusions. Against the diagnostic criteria of conviction and incorrigibility, the assumption that delusional beliefs are held with absolute certainty and are non-negotiable, I showed that July was willing to discuss her views, account for them and respond to challenges, following conversational rules. Against the criterion of implausibility, the assumption that delusional beliefs are false, I showed that while following common-sense assumptions and conversational conventions, issues of truth and falsity cannot be conversationally resolved. The implications of this approach for the diagnosis of delusions have been discussed elsewhere (Georgaca, 2000). I will now critically examine the position of this study with respect to the body of scientific and psychiatric knowledge it addresses and discuss the role of reflexivity in alternative modes of research on mental illness.

Deconstructing 'mental illness'

As I argued earlier, scientific facts are constructed and maintained by associations between groups of professionals and institutions. One of the prerequisites of the creation of facts is that their constructed character should be concealed. In this way they acquire the status of self-evident representations of external reality (Latour & Woolgar, 1979). 'Mental illness' has acquired the status of a fact through intense clinical and academic work over decades. It is these 'facts', reproduced by a series of associated practices, that have allowed psychiatry and clinical psychology to retain their powerful position in the management of human distress since the last century. We have argued elsewhere (Parker *et al.*, 1995) that non-pathologising research on mental illness would have to be based on a different view of language, a different theory of psychosis and alternative modes of research. Here, I have addressed the way that research practices based on reflexivity can provide the basis for non-pathologising inquiry into psychopathology. The 'fact' of 'mental illness' is produced by traditional research procedures in which the researcher assumes an unproblematic position of neutrality and the research findings are presented as if they were obtained by dispassionate and objective methods. An alternative mode of scientific research then, should not only acknowledge the constructive role of the researcher in designing and conducting their study, but also render that process explicit by describing and critically theorising the process of production of knowledge through it. The aim is not to unravel the 'truth' about mental illness, since that would reproduce objectivist assumptions, but rather to enable alternative theories and modes of research which, instead of normalising and pathologising, would change the types of questions to be asked and issues to be addressed, so that empowering research and practices on 'mental illness' can be developed. And, as I hope to have demonstrated, reflexivity should be at the core of such a project.

The conclusions drawn above, however, are not restricted to research on mental illness. Reflexivity, in my view, should be a central aspect of research in *any* subject area. Reflexive practice consists of *being aware of, and rendering visible, the constitutive role of the researcher in the production of the research findings and conclusions.* This applies to all stages of research, from research design to conducting, analysing and writing up the study. It also applies to all levels, from the micro-level of the researcher's interaction with participants to the macro-level of considering the place of the study in the existing bodies of knowledge and research.

Summary

In this chapter I have demonstrated some aspects of this reflexive procedure. Specifically, at the micro-level, I showed how the researcher as interviewer is actively implicated in the production of interview material. In a reflexive study, this not only has to be acknowledged but also explicitly illustrated through subjecting the interviewer's interventions to the same analysis as the interviewee's. At the macro-level, through showing that 'persecutory delusions' or 'auditory hallucinations' are not pre-existing facts but interactionally constructed and negotiated claims, I argued that reflexive analysis can reverse the effects of the objectivist modes of research which objectify and pathologise mental illness. It can open the way to empower those individuals with whom we are involved in the research.

In conclusion, whatever the field of research and the mode of reflexivity used, reflexivity is not something the researcher does retrospectively and writes up as a separate section. In truly reflexive research, reflexivity permeates and colours all aspects of the production and presentation of the study.

References

American Psychiatric Association (APA) (1994) *Diagnostic and Statistical Manual of Mental Disorders*, 4th edn. APA, Washington DC.

Banister, P., Burman, E., Parker I., Taylor, M. & Tindall, C. (1994) *Qualitative Methods in Psychology: A Research Guide*. Open University Press, Buckingham.

Barthes, R. (1987) The death of the author (translated by S. Heath). In *Image, Music, Text* (Heath, S., ed.). Fontana, London.

Burman, E. (1992) Identification and power in feminist therapy: a reflexive history of a discourse analysis. *Women's Studies International Forum*, **15**(4), 487–98.

Burr, V. (1995) *An Introduction to Social Constructionism*. Routledge, London.

Coulter, J. (1975) Perceptual accounts and interpretive asymetries. *Sociology*, **9**(3), 385–96.

Edwards, D. & Potter, J. (1992) *Discursive Psychology*. Sage Publications, London.

Gaines, A.D. (1992) From DSM-I to DSM-III-R; voices of self, mastery and the other: a cultural constructivist reading of US psychiatric classification. *Social Science and Medicine*, **35**, 3–24.

Georgaca, E. (1996) *Exploring 'Psychotic Discourse': The Construction and Negotiation of Reality and Subjectivity in Language*. PhD thesis, Manchester Metropolitan University.

Georgaca, E. (2000) Reality and discourse: a critical analysis of the category of 'delusions'. *British Journal of Medical Psychology*, **73**, 227–42.

Georgaca, E. (in press) Factualisation and plausibility in delusional discourse. *Philosophy, Psychiatry and Psychology*.

Goffman, E. (1981) *Forms of Talk*. Blackwell, Oxford.

Heritage, J.C. & Watson, D.R. (1979) Formulations as conversational objects. In *Everyday Language: Studies in Ethnomethodology* (Psathas, G., ed.). Irvington Publishers, New York.

Latour, B. & Woolgar, S. (1979) *Laboratory Life: The Social Construction of Scientific Facts*. Sage Publications, Beverly Hills.

Leudar, I. & Antaki, C. (1996a) Discourse participation, reported speech and research practices in social psychology. *Theory and Psychology*, **6**(1), 5–29.

Leudar, I. & Antaki, C. (1996b) Backing footing. *Theory and Psychology*, **6**(1), 41–6.

Mulkay, M. & Gilbert, G.N. (1985) Opening Pandora's box: A new approach to the sociological analysis of theory choice. *Knowledge and Society*, **5**, 113–39.

Myers, G. (1985) Texts as knowledge claims. *Social Studies of Science*, **15**, 593–630.

Parker, I. (1994) Reflexive research and the grounding of analysis: social psychology and the psy-complex. *Journal of Community and Applied Social Psychology*, **4**, 239–52.

Parker, I., Georgaca, E., Harper, D.J., McLaughlin, T. & Stowell-Smith, M. (1995) *Deconstructing Psychopathology*. Sage Publications, London.

Pollner, M. (1987) *Mundane Reason: Reality in Everyday and Sociological Discourse*. Cambridge University Press, Cambridge.

Potter, J. (1996a) *Representing Reality: Discourse, Rhetoric and Social Construction*. Sage Publications, London.

Potter, J. (1996b) Right and wrong footing. *Theory and Psychology*, **6**(1), 31–9.

Shotter, J. (1981) Telling and reporting: prospective and retrospective uses of self-ascriptions. In *The Psychology of Ordinary Explanations of Social Behaviour* (Antaki, C., ed.). Academic Press, London.

Wetherell, M. (1998) Positioning and interpretative repertoires: conversation analysis and post-structuralism in dialogue. *Discourse and Society*, **9**(3), 387–412.

CHAPTER 10

Reflexivity, 'bias' and the in-depth interview: developing shared meanings

Paula Nicolson

Positioning the self: author's story

As a health psychologist, I began using in-depth interviews and analysing the data qualitatively about fifteen years ago when there was very little psychological research of this kind to guide me, and even less enthusiasm within the discipline for such an approach. The inspiration and information on how to do qualitative research came from sociology – particularly symbolic interactionism and phenomenology.

In my case, the motivation came from my sense that mainstream studies of postnatal depression, my area of research, had little to contribute to *my* specific research questions. I had wanted to know how the women themselves *experienced* being depressed and how they explained the causes of their depression. I found one thing that I had not anticipated – namely the dynamic nature of the interview and data analysis processes in their own right. I discovered that the meaning of the participants' experiences was actively constructed through the interaction between the interviewer, participant and the situation itself. Conversations, I believe, are not neutral acts. In research the relationship between interviewer and participant, and the mutually understood meanings within that relationship, become an essential part of the data. Data analysis is further permeated with the researcher's *subjective reflections* relating to the experience of the interview and her or his retrospective analysis in the face of the data beyond the interpersonal context. I had previously been socialised to see this as a problem of 'bias'. Now I know there are different issues at stake.

Personal 'bias'?

My developing experience as a qualitative psychologist began in the early 1980s (when almost no psychologist would contemplate this kind of work) and continues twenty years later when qualitative research is generally tolerated if not wholeheartedly encouraged. Qualitative psychology though, is still a minority option both within the mainstream discipline and also (and perhaps, in particular) among those of us who work within or alongside clinicians and academics from other disciplines, particularly in the context of health services research. It is through experiences in this context that I have been drawn back many times to reflect upon the work I do and its value in the context of psychological research.

Research in psychology is different from, say, engineering research, in that the focus of the research is human behaviour, emotion, thoughts and experience and consequently the researcher has had some personal experience of the substantive research area. This applies equally to those who adopt a strict experimental method as to those who choose to do qualitative research. Some researchers, however, are more prepared than others to explore their relationship with their research area. As Judi Marshall explains:

> 'I have always chosen as research topics issues which have personal sig-
> nificance and which I need to explore in my own life.... This involvement
> provides the energy for research, heightens my potential as a sense maker
> and means that research has relevance to my life as a whole, not just my
> conceptual knowing' (1986, p. 194).

While it is likely that some traditional psychologists would dismiss Marshall's admission here as 'bias', a high level of personal commitment to research in this way would seem to play a vital part of any study for the reasons she suggests.

In this chapter, I focus on two studies – one on postnatal depression (PND), and the second on stress for staff working in neonatal intensive care units. Doing in-depth interviews in these two studies meant that my involvement in people's accounts of their lives became suffused with emotion and anxiety connected with their lives. This was made all the greater for me on occasions by the overriding need to make something of this data for both personal and academic purposes.

I had taken a risk collecting qualitative data in this way. The first time I did so, there were almost no precedents – certainly not in social psychology and not for psychologists drawing upon sociological ideas. On a personal level, I was interested in PND because I had been depressed during the year after my daughter's birth. While I had been quite clear it was because I did not like the role that accompanied motherhood – i.e. not working outside the home, being responsible for the domestic sphere and so on – the health visitor insisted I *had* PND. I knew I didn't *have* anything. I loved being a mother but I didn't want to be a housewife. I was thus, later, interested in why (if at all) other women found the postnatal period of their lives difficult and I was interested in them on a personal and on a scientific level. This could not be achieved through traditional methods available and acceptable to psychologists.

In the case of my second study, the risk of collecting qualitative data related to the expectations of colleagues and participants who (unlike most of the women in the PND study) saw themselves as being research-aware if not researchers in their own right. By this stage of my career, not only was qualitative psychology accepted (to a point) but I also felt more confident in taking a qualitative approach. This large-scale study of staff working in neonatal units was undertaken by a multidisciplinary team who worked well together. However, we also had a steering group that comprised two members in particular who had a virulent antipathy to qualitative research – one was a neonatologist and another a psychologist. They attacked everything I said, insisting that none of the participants would be prepared to be interviewed at length in the way I intended.

All this shook my confidence somewhat until I began to arrange and conduct the interviews. My respondents in fact engaged actively in the interviews – some with polite diligence but most with committed enthusiasm. The anxiety that the attacks on my approach to research raised, and the ensuing reflexivity, helped reinforce my confidence in qualitative research and the power of the in-depth interview.

Rowan (1981), describing some of the anxieties involved in doing research and making sense of what comes out of it, suggests that during the research process: 'Situations stir up anxieties and other feelings within the researcher, some of which may have much more to do with the researcher's own problems than anything going on out there in the world' (1981, p.77). It is essential, then, not only to acknowledge this but also to explore one's personal 'action' as a researcher in order to understand the research processes. One must also seek to recognise problems and anxieties related to this task and attempt to predict likely consequences.

In the case of my two research projects, as I got to know the respondents I came to feel a sense of involvement in, and obligation for, their well-being. This was reinforced by comments they made about the value of my visits for helping them let off steam and unburden themselves of certain anxieties. I was clearly an integral part of the research process for them. Although I wanted to publish the data, I also had to make a reassessment of what meaning the data actually had as it was being generated and thus to 'count in' the social process of constructing knowledge.

The views set out in this chapter derive from two qualitative research studies using in-depth interviews.[1] The first study was a longitudinal exploration of 24 women's experiences from pregnancy to around six months after childbirth, focusing on subjective accounts of depression (Nicolson, 1998). The second one was a cross-sectional study of the well-being of 45[2] health care staff in neonatal

---

[1] The methodologies employed in these studies are discussed in detail elsewhere (Nicolson, 1998; Tucker et al., 2001). In both cases an interview guide was developed, following Bott (1957) and Rapoport and Rapoport (1976). This aimed to understand how respondents justified and explained their own lives. The women in the first study were interviewed during pregnancy and then one, three and six months after the birth. The health care professionals in the neonatal units were interviewed once each over the course of a 12-month period at a mutually convenient time.

[2] There were 12 medical directors, 12 nursing directors and 21 middle-ranking and junior nurses and doctors interviewed.

intensive care units throughout the UK[3] (Tucker *et al.*, 2001). They were analysed using a hybrid interpretive framework comprising symbolic interactionist, phenomenological and psychodynamic perspectives (Nicolson, 1988).

Here, I look specifically at the research processes by examining the impact of the interview on the participants – an impact mediated by their relationship with myself as the interviewer. The expectation of a visit from a 'psychologist' stimulated reflexive contemplation in participants. There was a commonality in the way they reflected upon and constructed an analysis of their work and the role of motherhood, depression and/or stress in their lives. I suggest the ways in which the mutual engagement in the interview process enables a shared construction of meaning and experience through *reflexivity during, before and after the interviews*. Typically in psychology, the interview is not meant to have an impact, but to extract the 'truth' or 'facts' from the respondent about the subject matter in question. To have an impact introduces 'bias' and it is the central importance of this 'bias' for both constructing and revealing knowledge and understanding human psychology that underlies my research.

The two examples I draw on in this chapter demonstrate this and show how:

(1) The interviewer and the fact of being interviewed represent an *intervention* in the everyday life of the participant.
(2) The participants account for themselves and construct a *meaning* around 'self' in the context of motherhood and in the organisational context.

Analysing the data

The data from my interviews were analysed firstly through identification of themes, and then by attempting to identify conceptual issues relating to the substantive content of the research. In the first study, conducted at a time when there were few, if any, precedents in psychology, there was very little in the process of the data analysis that I would now call 'systematic'. I focused upon the answers to my research questions, particularly those related to how people experienced, described and accounted for depression, to provide the thematic analysis. Then, based upon reflexive reading of the transcripts and an attempt to understand the meaning of PND in the social context of motherhood, I developed a conceptual framework which has been discussed in detail elsewhere (Nicolson, 1988, 1998, 1999).

The neonatal study, begun in 1996, was part of a larger enterprise involving a team of statisticians, quantitative economists, health service researchers and clinical epidemiologists. Here, I put effort into demonstrating the 'science' in the

---

[3] I would like to acknowledge other key members of the neonatal staffing study research team, particularly Janet Tucker from the University of Aberdeen, and Gareth Parry and Chris McCabe from the University of Sheffield.

qualitative psychology element of the study. To do this, I generated the list of participants from a stratified sample. The identification of themes was carried out 'objectively', and independently, by myself and a colleague who was not otherwise involved in the project. The themes were illustrated via the evidence of brief quotations and were included as a chapter in the report.

The conceptual issues which related to telling of the experience of working in a highly stressed environment were excluded from the formal research report as 'surplus to requirements'. After reflection, however, I sensed the lifelessness of the approach taken by the team (including myself). I began to think again about the problem of being a qualitative psychologist in a traditional setting. As Sampson (1993) puts it:

> 'Proponents of this dominant tradition have been so insistent on searching for the essential qualities housed within the individual that they have created *two* conceptual dilemmas for themselves ... The first involves the investigators' failure to pay attention to their own activities; the second involves their failure to attend closely to their subjects' activities' (p.18).

Reflexivity in action: the interview

I now present brief extracts from both studies to indicate the ways in which meaning is constructed, how the in-depth research interview represents an intervention and how the process of the interview itself generates a biography or history for the participants. My argument is that this constitutes valid data and that through counting the reflexive and subjective elements of the engagement between the research participants some important psychological questions can be addressed.

Reflexivity in qualitative research has been defined in a number of ways (for instance, see Doherty, 2000). For those engaged in symbolic interactionist, feminist, postmodern or social constructionist projects, it continues to be a highly contentious but key concept (see Banister *et al.*, 1994). In the research interview, reflexivity requires an analytic approach that accounts for and respects 'the different meanings brought to the research by researcher and volunteer' (Parker, cited in Banister *et al.*, 1994, p.14). This assumes the potential for the shared understanding of events or emotional experience. It also assumes that the participants experience a sense of meaning prior to the research encounter. Alternatively, it may be used to confirm a relativist position, i.e. that talk between respondent and interviewer is functional in creating what might be seen as individual, prior experiences and meanings. As Steier puts it, 'taking reflexivity seriously in doing research is marked by a concern for recognising that constructing is a social process, rooted in language, not located inside one's head' (1991, p.5).

Used in this way reflexivity assumes an individual with a biography and a dynamic sense of her or his life's meaning (Nicolson, 1995, 1998).[4] The interview itself is the site of far more activity than simply the collection of verbal data. It is a reflexive process and one in which a relationship is established. This relationship becomes almost a *third actor* in the research scenario.[5]

The interview itself develops a biography and a history – it exists across time, anticipating the future encounter, capturing the present and reflecting the past relationship. The biographical and historical characteristics of the interview are most pronounced when they are repeated as in a longitudinal study. This was the case with the PND interviews, in which several respondents were interviewed on four occasions. Between each visit (and before the first one) the participants and I had specific thoughts, feelings, expectations and reflections on what the interview would mean and how the experience would impact upon the interaction between us and upon our lives.

My concern on one level was to ensure that data was collected and that it was both useful and useable. I was also concerned about the way I would be perceived and about the experiences that would be revealed. The content of both studies involved distress at different levels and this had its impact upon me (questioning and listening) and the respondent (telling and remembering). In order to focus on the impact that events and experiences have upon the lives of the respondent, the researcher necessarily has to understand and 'get to know' the person they are interviewing. Shedding my sense of being an 'objective' researcher, I found I cared about the people I was interviewing – some more than others, of course. I developed a feeling of being responsible for their pain and happiness that was not totally inappropriate given the level of intimate revelations that took place. However, such notions are anathema in traditional psychology, and it takes reflexive awareness to recognise their existence.

These points, and the multiple layers surrounding reflexivity, subjectivity and bias in the interview, are best illustrated through examples. In the extract below (Box 10.1), Jane tells of her growing sense of 'self' as a mother and of the kind of mother she feels she is. From what she says, this reflexivity appears to be the direct result of being a participant in the interview: a reflexive stance to identity and change that is present throughout the extract.

Michael, a senior doctor participating in the neonatal staffing study, also uses the experience of being interviewed to talk to and for himself (as well as to me) about his 'self' and reflect upon the dilemmas he currently faces (Box 10.2). Not

---

[4] For example, in my research interviews I always ended by asking the respondent how they had found the experience. Frequently in response to this or to other questions they will say 'I hadn't seen it that way before' or 'Talking about it clarified . . .'.

[5] These ideas were developed initially by symbolic interactionist and phenomenological psychologists in the 1940s–1960s (mostly) in the USA. Some of these ideas influenced the social psychology of the 1970s–1980s and the epistemology of contemporary qualitative psychologies, particularly aspects of discourse analysis (e.g. Harré & Secord, 1972).

Box 10.1   Being reflexive about identity change

Jane: I used to see my friend sit there and play bricks and imagine things with her two boys and I'd think 'how boring'. I thought I would think the same thing when I had a baby. I thought it'd be the same as before. It's not. I've changed in that way. I enjoy this sitting and playing. To see her [the baby] smiling and laughing and everything – it's different to how I thought in the beginning. *You don't realise how much you've changed until you talk about it like this* [my emphasis].

Box 10.2   Stress of balancing job and family roles

Michael: My parents see my achievements as being important . . . It all looks great to them . . . but . . . the reality is – when I am asked 'how's work?' – my comment was 'Stressful! It's rewarding but stressful'. I wouldn't give it up. I wouldn't resign my job – it's rewarding – but it's stressful. My biggest fear, I suppose, is that that stress will take its toll on me and my family – I would feel very cheated if that happened. I try to deal with it – I am not bad at it – I have colleagues who hang around until all hours.
Paula: But that is a way of avoiding facing their families, isn't it?
M: Do you think so?
P: Absolutely.

---

only does he feel alone in the working context, but he also has to live up to his sense of how others (he believes) see him. In this example, he identifies the 'others' as his parents, and his immediate family of wife and children.

This extract highlights my involvement with the stress Michael experiences as he seeks to balance job and family and with his fears about how he (as compared to his colleagues) handles the stress. I engage him in a somewhat therapeutic manner. I was surprised about this when I listened to the tape after the interview and read the transcript. The interview had shifted ground, almost without me realising, from information gathering to a quite intimate discussion of Michael's experiences and how he should make sense of them. The reason for this shift may become clearer later in this chapter. As I write this, two years after the only occasion I met him, I wonder whether Michael managed to resolve the fierce conflicts in his life and hope that our meeting gave him clues about how to tackle his stressful life.

Each encounter between researcher and participant, irrespective of the individuals involved or the duration of the research, exists in a number of dimensions. Mead's (1934) work on the self as subject and object promotes understanding of how an interview is not simply a means of collecting qualitative data on tape for subsequent analysis. Talking to another human being brings individual and shared consciousness into play. Reflexive, discursive and unconscious dimensions are part of the encounter. For the interviewer, there are the multiple anxieties about whether and how the encounter will work. Will rapport be established? Will the respondent have anything of substance to say? Will the questions be both well-constructed and well-received?

Thinking about the interview retrospectively gives both respondent and interviewer more time for reflexivity. The interviewer will have the tape and transcript to focus on as well as the memory of certain aspects of the encounter and the 'atmosphere'. The respondent will have the memory of their thoughts and emotions generated by the interview process and their relationship with the interviewer.

Constructing the research relationship

My decision to examine the importance of the research interview itself for the production of knowledge (about postnatal depression and the experience of working in a stressful environment) arose during the process of analysing the tape-recorded interviews. It became clear that the relationship between interviewer and respondent was a dynamic, developing one. Most respondents gave thought in advance to what they would say at the meeting, and for the first set of participants (in the PND study) this was also done between interview sessions. In other words, the process of being a respondent produced a long-term self-conscious reflexivity. Respondents engaged with the interviewer in a complex reflexive process, which had implications for the meaning and understanding of the data and of the experience itself.

The process, then, raises important theoretical issues about the way individuals attribute and reflect upon the meaning of experience and subjectivity-identity. The research interview is part of a process of knowledge production – about both subjectivity and the substantive content of the interview. In particular, two aspects of the research relationship emerged from examination of the data produced in this way:

- The researcher–respondent interactions as a *dynamic social process*.
- The related *production of subjectivity* as both 'I'/'Me' (i.e. immediate consciousness/self as subject and reflexive consciousness/self as object), both in anticipation of the interview period and during its course.

Researcher–respondent interactions: the interview as intervention

The relationship between interviewer and respondent built up its own momentum. The interviews themselves were perceived to be helpful, even therapeutic, a reality underlined by the comments of several respondents and the fact that so few of them dropped out. As Angela, a participant in the PND study, told me, 'I find it really helpful to talk, especially when I feel depressed and frustrated. I said to my friend, "My psychiatrist is coming tomorrow." If you hadn't been coming I would have got depressed.'

Angela had been interviewed on two previous occasions and had a clear sense of what she both expected and experienced during and between the interviews. In the neonatal staffing study, which was neither explicitly about mood or emotion nor longitudinal in structure, there was still a sense from several participants that they had looked forward to the opportunity to unburden themselves, to talk over some work-related matters of concern. Michael, a participant in a senior and responsible position, and thus professionally isolated, told me he had 'looked forward to this discussion – there are issues here that I want to sort out because I am not seriously depressed or deranged'.

Talking about emotional issues is not integral to the culture with which Michael – as a man and a doctor – is most familiar. He needed to distinguish between talking to a psychologist on a professional, clinical level and having a conversation with a researcher he knew to be a psychologist. He seemed to associate the former with an admission to himself of emotional disturbance, while taking advantage of the latter type of encounter was apparently acceptable to him. The content of the encounter had similarities with a clinical or counselling interview and this content was constructed as part of the process of our mutual engagement. This type of research becomes, inevitably, a form of intervention (see Coyle & Wright, 1996) in that it demands a reflexive consciousness from both participants. It also enables the expression of feelings and ideas in confidence without the fear of 'diagnosis' or upsetting others by expressing anxieties or antagonisms.

Constructing the meaning of self

The examples discussed above cannot be seen as separate from the process of constructing a sense of selfhood through talk. This is a dynamic and ongoing process in almost any relationship but particularly in one where emotion, behaviour and personal experience are the focus of the encounter. In the example that follows (Box 10.3) Norma, a midwife, reveals her ambivalence about becoming a mother through the process of talking to me.

The extract in Box 10.3 represents the start of a process stimulated by the interview. For Norma, focusing upon her fear of personal change as her pregnancy advances becomes inevitable. She shifts away from the potential pleasures and personal growth that a having a baby might mean and considers whether or not a baby is the end of 'self' or whether it is possible to live beyond the arrival of the baby to get to the other side. She divides 'mother' from 'person'. She has a view of what a 'good mother' is and does. The good mother gives herself up to the baby, while a good person is exemplified by herself as she is now and by her non-mother friends. The good person is independent and free. That independence is so separate from the mother that Norma believes that becoming a mother will bring

> ## Box 10.3 Ambivalence and shifting positions
>
> *Norma:* I kind of thought that if I have a baby, that's the end of me as a person. I'd never be able to do anything again and I suppose one of my sisters is a single mother and she's gone on to university. And she was very supportive . . . and said 'there's life afterwards!' I think that helped a lot.
>
> *Paula:* What made you think that way?
>
> *N:* Well, I don't know. I don't have many friends who have babies. The women I work with have babies. I just look after women and babies for seven days and then they go back into the community. But you see women on buses with pushchairs – and I think of my own experience of my own mother. She was a midwife and gave up work to have children and her whole life revolved around us. I felt that – it's a very Irish thing I suppose – but to be a good mother I'd have to be at home all the time to really give myself. And I just liked to have my freedom, and as I say most of my friends are very independent. And I thought . . . well they won't want to know me. My friends won't want to be around me and a crying baby. You go to a party and there's a woman with a baby. In a way she is excluded. She ends up running after the baby – feeding, changing it. It's different you know. I was very frightened. I thought this is it. I'm just going to come to a stop and I didn't think I'd be able to organise myself enough to do all the things I wanted to do.

about her rejection by her peer group. There is a clear implication of self-rejection here also. Norma constructed her sense of herself as a mother as she sees motherhood rather than in any way related to herself going through a life stage of (relatively) normal human development.

Both Mead (1934) and Lacan (1949) have suggested a model of self and subjectivity that is preceded by the social order. Subjectivity is structured through gaining entry into the social world by taking a place in the symbolic order. Although self and subjectivity are not wholly fixed in either author's version, Lacan stresses the production of subjectivity through discursive relations and the centrality of language in consciousness and self-awareness which is within the terms set by pre-existing social relations and cultural values. Lacan theorises subjectivity in a way that enables resistance to the inherent subordination of women (see Urwin, 1984) but leads to the conclusion that subjectivity cannot transcend the existing pattern of social and discursive relations.

The example in Box 10.4 shows Michael's awareness of the pre-existing role he fills in the organisation and in relation to being a husband and father. He measures himself against his understanding of how these roles fit into the social structure and evaluates himself and his performance in accordance with standards he sees as being set outside himself. He sees these standards as more important for self-evaluation than his own judgements about what is possible for him. Yet, when attempting to evaluate his role in these contexts, he experiences such difficulties that his speech eventually fades out.

> ## Box 10.4 Evaluating role performance
>
> *Michael:* My problem is that I feel that I am failing in both departments – I am not particularly succeeding in work because I try to get home – and I am not particularly succeeding at home because I am not really that efficient at home – I feel I am doing a mediocre job. Sometimes I wish I could do a really good job in one.
>
> *Paula:* Have you told your wife that – the way you have told me?
>
> *M:* Yes – we talk a lot – some of it you can't blame on work – she certainly feels that . . . we are on a bit of a knife edge at the moment – I feel – I hope it works; I am optimistic but I just can't seem to manage it all you know – I would love to do a good job here – but if I do a good job here I seem to need to be here all the time – I don't want to be here all the time – I have no desire to . . .

Examining the transcripts revealed an ongoing dialogue which, at the practical level, was part of a getting-to-know process through which the respondent managed self-presentation to the interviewer. However, this was tied to discursive and unconscious levels of knowledge.

There is also evidence of how the interview encourages the relating of self to context and also the dynamic re-production of self through reflexivity. Angela (Box 10.5) refers to conversations with others and her ongoing account of herself to me, to focus on the contradictions of her changing self-consciousness (ME/ discursive consciousness opposed to her I/subjective/practical consciousness). There are also indicators of the unconscious present in her transcripts which represent the link between the contradictory facets of subjectivity (ideas discussed in Giddens' (1979) theory of structuration).

> ## Box 10.5 Contradictory facets of subjectivity
>
> *Angela:* I was saying to my friend the other day 'I can't understand why my memory is just going! It used to be so good'. I suppose it's because of the job I was doing. I'd remember numbers, faces, addresses – my memory was really spot on. And now, I'm just as bad as my mum – which is something I vowed I'd never ever be. It always used to annoy me when my mum was so forgetful. I remember getting very cross with her at times. Now I'm doing exactly the same thing.

Thus, she says: 'I can't understand why my memory is just going' (practical consciousness/I). She reflects upon why she is so concerned (i.e. her previous skills and her fear of being as her mother seems to be.) She also talks of herself as having a 'lack of routine' – she is lost behind the children, just as her memory is lost. She is actively becoming something she does not wish to be. Because she cannot explain these contradictions, she deals with them by saying later in the interview: 'I think it's just me'.

Summary

The processes involved in the in-depth interview are not (and can never be) neutral, objective and unbiased acts: interviewer and respondent are engaging (or failing to engage) with each other. As this process involves a mutual construction of the topics under discussion, *both participants need to be reflexive.*

Taking a qualitative approach to psychological research via the in-depth interview has important implications for both researcher and respondent. Conducting a survey or experiment may generate compelling findings but the focus will remain upon the data and the theoretical framework. The in-depth interview, by contrast, requires *commitment* to the life of the participant. The researcher needs to continually reflect on the research by 'staying with' the participant through the process of co-constructing their relationship.

References

Banister, P., Burman, E., Parker, I.,Taylor, M. & Tindall, C. (1994) *Qualitative Methods in Psychology: A Research Guide.* Open University Press, Buckingham.

Bott, E. (1957) *Family and Social Network.* Tavistock, London.

Coyle, A. & Wright, C. (1996) Using the counselling interview to collect research data on sensitive topics. *Journal of Health Psychology,* 1(4), 431–40.

Doherty, K. (2000) *Going it Alone: A Discursive Psychological Analysis of Identity and Enterprise Culture.* PhD thesis, University of Sheffield.

Giddens, A. (1979) *Central Problems in Social Theory.* Macmillan, Basingstoke.

Harré, R. & Secord, P.F. (1972) *The Explanation of Social Behaviour.* Blackwell, Oxford.

Henwood, K. & Nicolson, P. (1995) Qualitative research. *The Psychologist,* 8(3), 456–7.

Lacan, J. (1949) The mirror stage as formative of the function of the 'I' in psychoanalytic experience. In *Ecrits: A Selection.* Routledge, London.

Marshall, J. (1986) Exploring the experiences of women managers: towards a rigour in qualitative methods. In *Feminist Social Psychology: Developing Theory and Practice* (Wilkinson, S.J., ed.). Open University Press, Milton Keynes.

Mead, G.H. (1934) *Mind, Self and Society.* University of Chicago Press, Chicago.

Nicolson, P. (1988) *The Social Psychology of 'Postnatal Depression'.* PhD thesis, University of London (LSE).

Nicolson, P. (1995) Qualitative research and mental health: analyzing subjectivity. *Journal of Mental Health,* 4(4), 337–45.

Nicolson, P. (1998) *Postnatal Depression: Psychology, Science and the Transition to Motherhood.* Routledge, London.

Nicolson, P. (1999) Loss, happiness and postpartum depression: the ultimate paradox. *Canadian Psychology,* 40(2), 162–78.

Parker, I. (1994) Qualitative research. In *Qualitative Methods in Psychology: A Research Guide* (Banister, P., Burman, E., Parker, I.,Taylor, M. & Tindall, C., eds). Open University Press, Buckingham.

Rapoport, R. & Rapoport, R. (1976) *Dual Career Families Revisited*. Martin Robertson, Oxford.

Rowan, J. (1981) From anxiety to method in the behavioural sciences. In *Human Inquiry: A Sourcebook of New Paradigm Research* (Reason, P. & Rowan, J., eds). Wiley, Chichester.

Sampson, E.E. (1993) *Celebrating the Other: A Dialogue of Human Nature*. Harvester Wheatsheaf, London.

Steier, F. (1991) *Research and Reflexivity*. Sage Publications, London.

Tucker, J., Parry, G., McCabe, C. & Nicolson, P. (2001) *United Kingdom Neonatal Staffing Study. Health Technology Assessment*. NHS Executive, Southampton.

Urwin, K. (1984) Power relations and emergence of language. In *Changing the Subject* (Henriques, J., Hollway, W., Urwin, C., Venn, C. & Walkerdine, V., eds). Methuen, London.

CHAPTER 11

Shifting researcher positions during a group interview study: a reflexive analysis and re-view

Brendan Gough

Positioning the self: author's story

I've been working as a 'critical social psychologist' for eight years now, doing qualitative research in the area of men and masculinities. Mostly I have used discourse analysis to examine material from group discussions with men, and have published work on contemporary masculinities, sexism and homophobia. Theoretically, I am influenced by both social constructionist and psychoanalytic writing, and the interface between these two traditions. With this in mind, I am critical of definitions and practices around reflexivity which presume a conscious subject with unproblematic access to inner 'intentions', 'motivations', 'feelings' – we cannot know fully what prompts us to choose a particular research project, to ask certain questions, to respond in specific ways, etc. How can we pin down a self which is multi-faceted, dynamic and embedded in language and social relationships? Consequently, reflexive analysis must be re-viewed as similarly complex and tenuous – a way of increasing the visibility of diverse, contradictory positions while simultaneously acknowledging the constructed quality of such a project (see Steier, 1991).

This chapter argues that researcher contributions to research interviews can entail manifold, and sometimes contradictory, positions and serve different functions. To illustrate this, I present a range of examples of researcher intervention during a group interview study with male university students. By subjecting interview transcripts to critical scrutiny, the multifarious, shifting and occasionally unintended positions adopted by the interviewer come into view, and an impression of researcher subjectivity as complex and difficult to control emerges. As well as underlining contemporary notions of selfhood as variable and dynamic, I suggest that an analysis of researcher involvement within interview texts facilitates effective reflexive qualitative research.

Introduction

This chapter looks back on a group interview project I conducted in 1995, with a specific focus on how I, as the researcher, intervened in the interviews. I contend that close scrutiny of researcher talk, and how this is taken up by participants, can form a useful part of a broader reflexive project, as it helps to identify the adoption of practices which the researcher may never have intended. The activity of examining researcher talk in conjunction with participant talk helps to illuminate the co-construction of data in qualitative research settings. With this in mind, I first reconsidered the 1995 data four years later and produced a conference paper (Gough, 1999), which forms the basis of this chapter. But for present purposes I have also added another layer of reflexivity using a rhetorical device, which I call the 'Reflexive Voice' (RV), which contributes further reflections in 2002 to those provided in 1999. The use of such devices highlights the many voices which can be brought to bear on research data and is common in postmodern texts (see Stainton-Rogers *et al.*, 1995; Seale, 1999; Denzin, 2001).

The study

To facilitate reflexivity, it is important to be 'transparent', i.e. to provide as much information as possible about the steps involved in the research project, including details about how the topic was selected, how participants were recruited, which methods were used as well as research outcomes (transcripts, analysis etc.). Before considering the interview transcripts, the research on which this chapter is based is contextualised.

The project which forms the basis of this chapter was the original (1995) study, which prompted a wider, ongoing programme of research – the Men, Masculinities and Discourse project (see Gough, 1998). Briefly, the aim of the study was to explore issues around masculine identities by examining heterosexual men's talk in a university setting, with a view to exploring the implications for gender relations. This work can be located within a critical/feminist social psychology framework and, as such, is concerned to highlight problems of discourses and practices around masculinity which are used to subordinate 'others', such as women and gay men (e.g. Gough & Edwards, 1998; Wetherell & Edley, 1999). Such research is informed by and addresses a wider cultural context in which boys and men are popularly construed variously as 'lost', 'confused', 'at risk', 'vulnerable' ... (compared to the newly 'empowered' woman – see Skelton, 1998). For example, recent debates within the UK education sector have stressed the need to tackle boys' 'under-achievement' at school compared with that of girls (Raphael-Reed, 1999). Yet such debates play down or ignore men's continued access to power (and women's experiences of powerlessness). Further, they treat men as a homogenous group, thereby neglecting relations and differences of class, race, ethnicity, (dis)ability, sexuality etc. Work in critical/feminist social psychology attempts to make explicit the operation of power by interrogating men's talk and practices.

Recent publications, for example, have critically examined men's talk which presents gender difference and male superiority in terms of 'nature' (i.e. men are 'naturally' different from or superior to women because of genetics, hormones, evolution etc.) or even 'liberal' values (i.e. where the male speaker presents himself as tolerant before producing a statement widely regarded as prejudiced, as in 'I'm not sexist but ... women shouldn't be allowed to fly planes.') (see Gill, 1993; Gough, 1998). So, I approached the research from the perspective of a critical qualitative researcher and psychologist interested in examining how men constructed self and other(s) and contextualising this within broader cultural discourses around gender relations in contemporary society.

The particular 1995 study under scrutiny here comprised three group discussions with second-level male psychology students (average number three plus researcher), recruited from class upon request for volunteers. The discussions were not part of any course requirements. The mean age of the white, heterosexual participants was 23 and all were from the north of England, with many presenting themselves as having working-class origins. A semi-structured 'polite interrogation' approach was adopted to gather data on the participants' views on issues regarding gender and sexuality whereby main topics (relationships, sport, college, work etc.) were gently explored and probed. Discussions lasting on average 1.5 hours were recorded, transcribed and subjected to a Foucauldian-inspired discourse analysis of the kind advocated by Parker (1994) and Willott and Griffin (1997).

Post-hoc reflexivity

The section heading reflects my return to the transcripts some four years later (1999), a re-view of how the data was produced and examined. Quite possibly this is a belated attempt to atone for what now looks like fairly un-reflexive qualitative research! In addition, I inject another layer of reflexivity from the present moment (2002), a 'reflexive voice' (RV) which disrupts the narrative of the chapter at key points in order to develop or question my initial reflexive analysis. This reflexive voice is written in a broadly psychoanalytic register, since I have recently been swayed by psychoanalytic accounts of (masculine) subjectivities (see Gough, in press). For present purposes, psychoanalytic (particularly Kleinian) concepts, such as anxiety and projection, can help explain the various positions I took up in the group discussions.

Reconsidering my general semi-structured interview approach in the discussions (see Smith, 1995), I seemed interested to follow participant talk as it developed and produced themes unanticipated by the questions I had prepared. Indeed, my opening spiel to each group emphasised their active participation, with the following phrases typically deployed: 'I want it to be as laid back as possible'; 'I've a few topics I'd like to pursue but I don't want to restrict the conversation unnaturally, so if other things come up we'll just follow those, OK?'. But this approach still implies a traditional relationship between researcher and participant, with the researcher remaining fairly detached, apart from supplying questions (the 'polite interrogator') and 'allowing' some deviation from script, and the participants treated as separate, reactive, data givers. Such a relationship is structured by my asking specific questions, such as: 'What does it mean to be a man? Would you consider yourselves to be "new men"? What are your thoughts on homosexuality?' In addition, these questions would be followed up with the usual prompts, such as 'Can you give me any examples . . . ? In what ways . . . ? Why do you think that is?'

RV: 'Yes, this facilitating stance which encourages participant rather than researcher talk seems borne of defence – it is a safe, contained position which protects against role uncertainty and which avoids personal disclosure by the researcher. Ironically, a very "masculine" position featuring self-control and detachment.'

Yet, from re-reading the transcripts of the research, it became apparent that I adopted a variety of positions beyond this questioning role at different points. In general, I seemed to oscillate between being detached from, and involved in, the talk. When I did enter the conversation, I did so in a variety of ways, such as asking questions but also making comments on particular statements, presenting criticism of certain views, attempting humorous remarks and deflecting questions directed at me. Upon reviewing these positions in context, it strikes me that I was struggling to manage two main conflicts and identities. Firstly, I seemed to oscillate between the presumed stance of the detached polite interrogator restricted to asking questions, and the involved co-participant interested in contributing to the conversations. Secondly, talk perceived as 'problematic' in some way (sexist, homophobic etc.) by myself as the researcher I either ignored or attempted to challenge – there seemed to be no fixed or predictable response. Instead of merely collecting data, then, I was engaged in diverse and conflicting negotiations with participants, unforeseen when the research was first conceived and conducted. The analysis which follows aims to contextualise, understand and evaluate these various instances of researcher (in-)activity within the texts, and problems of reflexive practice which rely on an image of a unitary, knowing researcher. The following categories of researcher intervention are now discussed: researcher as 'pundit', 'comedian', 'critic' and 'professional'.

Researcher as 'pundit'

As well as asking questions and using prompts, there were occasions when my intervention may have been more self-indulgent or narcissistic. This came across most strongly when I summarised or reflected back statements provided by the participants. It occurs to me that such interventions resemble those offered by sports commentators and panelists ('pundits') who perhaps articulate what the 'ordinary' fan thinks, albeit with typically more jargon. Consider the following extract – the conversation up to this point had been about masculinity as aggressive and explosive, a notion which Sam challenges:

Sam: I've seen a lot of women that will lose their cool quite quickly.
Interviewer: But is that not another dimension to masculinity, this idea of being cool and rational?
Glen: Yeah, because men don't – I think women make a lot of noise and don't do anything . . .

Here is an example of the researcher weighing in with an unplanned comment on a participant's statement, perhaps heard as 'authoritative', as agreement is forthcoming (from Glen) – an agreement which may not have been gleaned had I remained quiet. So, the researcher gets involved, but not really on a personal level. A more personal comment might have involved me giving examples from my experience of men or myself assuming a cool poise (or even countering with examples of women being cool) and confirming that notion of masculinity rather than directing my observation back to participants as a question. Assuming this role of summariser is perhaps not surprising in the light of how (most) research contexts are framed by disciplinary and institutional parameters within which participants may feel uncomfortable or 'naïve', and where the researcher is seen as an authority figure (see Ballinger & Payne, 2000). On this point it is pertinent to remind ourselves of my lecturing position: these research participants were also my students. Could my intervention in the text be a case of the researcher taking advantage of status in order to influence or structure the talk?

> *RV:* 'Well, possibly. It certainly looks like an academic rather than a personal intervention, very "cool and rational" in fact! In speaking about masculinity in this way, I effectively enact this very version of masculinity, this suppression of the personal. Perhaps (unconsciously) I was exploring my own masculinity through the participants' words – they were discussing ideas and issues that were personally relevant for me as a young man, but possibly unresolved. Maintaining an academic posture concentrates my gaze on others and upholds the contained, secure, powerful position of the research facilitator.'

Nonetheless, we must not overestimate the power of the researcher to dictate; participants can and do resist the researcher's interpretations, as the following extract demonstrates:

Jack: I think things are probably changing now due to all the heavy industries, gettin' laid off, it gets a bit more service-orientated where women can compete on a man's level because it's not physical any more.

Interviewer: Yeah.

Jack: Skills, as opposed to just brute force in certain jobs.

I: That's what I was going to mention – we live in a post-industrial society where manufacturing industry has diminished and with feminism and other social changes the traditional bases of authority for men have been threatened, I mean, any comments on that?

Glen: Is it threatened though? It may be for older people who've had that but I didn't have that in the first place. I've just come along and it's as it is and you just take it as it is. I don't say 'back in Victorian times I could've done this'.

I: What about in relationships with women – partners and friends?

My re-iteration of Jack's construction of contemporary gender relations in the labour market uses academic language ('post-industrial' etc.) and, perhaps realising my departure from the researcher's role as questioner, this comment is rendered as a question at the end of the utterance. But my characterisation is clearly challenged by Glen in the next turn, who locates men as threatened by social change in an older generation. Perhaps surprised, perhaps irritated by such 'insubordination', I move to change the subject slightly at the earliest opportunity (on to relationships). The researcher's 'authoritative' view is evidently open to question.

> *RV:* 'Hmmm, the researcher's paternal wisdom is undermined, destabilised and is hastily restored through re-establishing the questioning role, and with it, familiar power relations. There is an avoidance of debate, a reluctance to engage with Glen on this issue, which serves to protect me against potential uncertainty and tension associated with unanticipated (and therefore unplanned) discussion. I must not have felt very secure in my researcher role and so opted for control and closure rather than engagement and openness, thereby missing out on potentially very interesting data!'

Researcher as 'comedian'

Deploying 'humorous' remarks was another departure from merely asking questions:

Jack: . . . people look to label because it makes them feel safer, like to label . . . they think they know where they stand and they can control, but it's a lot more complex. . . .

Interviewer: Psychologists are the worst offenders! [group laughter].

J: Yeah.

Glen: The media, *The Guardian* and psychologists on Channel 4! [group laughter].

I suppose the use of humour helps to suggest the illusion of 'normal' conversation, with the researcher temporarily colluding as one of the 'lads', albeit in this case one limited to brief interjections. This particular example could indicate a degree of self-deprecation, perhaps in an effort to reduce power differentials or, perhaps more likely, to create distance between myself and (the maligned) psychologists, hence appearing liberal or sophisticated (either way attempting to endear myself to the participants, as indicated by participants' laughter and further endorsement by Glen). Perhaps such occasional contributions give the impression of participation, thus rendering, temporarily, the otherwise peculiar position of polite interrogator less salient.

> RV: 'It is also possible that humour is attempted as a defence in the light of anxiety or discomfort around my "difference" (as researcher, tutor, outsider) and "using" the participants for data. Humour enables a temporary alliance to be forged so that difference is momentarily erased. By contributing to and encouraging this "banter" within the group, am I perhaps seeking to assuage guilt, to reassure myself that, if nothing else, the participants at least derive some enjoyment from their participation?'

Hence, it is difficult to pinpoint exactly why certain interventions were made – and the intentions read into these by the participants themselves – making for a rather fraught reflexive endeavour.

Other strategies I adopted include self-disclosure, done, of course, in a humorous way:

Sam: I know a lot of women who would say 'Look at shoes' and like three weeks later it'll be 'I've got enough money now'.
Interviewer: I'd be like that! [group laughter].
Jack: Women think about what they're wearing – they'll shop, think about how they look as opposed to [men] paying a logo that tells everybody how...
I: I still go for brand names!

Such admissions on the part of the researcher again bolster the image of apparent participation, presenting the researcher as human or out of role by virtue of identifying with derogated other(s) – in this case the determined female shoe shopper and the shallow male label fiend.

> RV: 'I think also I may have been attempting to query the casual association between women and shopping presented initially by Sam, because it is stereotypical and because I knew that many men enjoyed shopping – like myself, as I then claim. So, is this a case of personal investment in "modern" constructions of femininity and masculinity which emphasise multiplicity and complexity? What Stainton-Rogers *et al.* (1995) call the "People Like Us" syndrome, whereby the researcher (unwittingly) designs and interprets research which confirms their own beliefs and values?'

Researcher as 'critic': confronting 'problematic' participant talk

But what if the researcher is tempted to respond to participant talk which she or he considers problematic in some way? This is a real dilemma, which again places stress on the researcher's questioning role. Upon re-reading the transcripts, it appears that I avoid commenting on some issues but not others. Often when something was said which I consider sexist or homophobic, I don't intervene because there was an interesting discussion in full swing between the participants (hence the promise of 'juicy' data). Moreover, sometimes other participants challenged the speaker in much the same way as I might have done:

Tom: Calling women 'birds', uhh [exasperation]. God, the stress I get for that, sometimes say it in the wrong place

John: It is degrading though.

T: It's not, it's....

J: I, I wouldn't call, well you know that, don't you?

T: Yeah, but callin' them birds it's not like that, I mean a bird is like a nice little, cheepy little, you know, bird, it's sweet and has a nice voice....

J: Sits beside you when you want it [T laughs] but when you want it to fly away just....

T: Back in the cage!

J: [ironic] That's not sexist at all, is it?

I remember enjoying this exchange, absolved from responding and appreciating the richness of the dialectic.

> *RV:* 'Yes, just listening rather than intervening proved very relaxing, and also exciting – the transgressions of the other (Tom) fairly titillating, expressing "taboo" sentiments. Perhaps echoing the pleasure of the "voyeur", removed from the action but all-seeing?'

When making a critical contribution myself, humour again proved a useful way of framing so as not to undermine or subordinate the participant's position seriously or directly:

Mal: When women get to about 50 years old, there's that emptiness, they get that broodiness again, don't they? And I think they actually like that mothering....

Jack: Yeah, I mean some of it has a biological basis to it....

Interviewer: That's not what feminists say! [Group laughter].

In this case, the objection is attributed to a vague, external, homogenous 'other' ('feminists') rather than myself, thereby minimising any discomfort for me and the participants. An abandonment of academic insights about the complex differences and debates between feminisms is evident here in favour of partial collusion and gentle critique. In fact, it appears that most of my critical interventions

are reserved for intimations of biological determinism applied to gender difference, a perspective which I tend to reject from a social constructionist position
which regards gender and the body as mediated through culture (see Gough,
1998).

> RV: 'A case of having my cake and eating it — a comment which desires simul-
> taneous closeness to and distance from the participants? Expressing my
> ambivalence: on the one hand managing the interaction as a researcher, on the
> other wanting to "join in with the lads" as a fellow male.'

On a few occasions, however, my critique was more direct:

Sam: They're finding now that male homosexuals have got a slightly smaller
hippocampus, so they've been born with a woman's sexuality if you like. . . .
Interviewer: But is having a differently sized hippocampus necessarily equal to
sexuality?
S: If there was a definite correlation and it carried on to be shown that 99% of
homosexuals did have corresponding sized hippocampuses then I would be
interested in the results. . . .
I: But even if that were true it doesn't mean that sexuality follows from that. . . .
Glen: There's a lot of gay men who get married and have kids and try to convince
themselves that they're not and then years later . . . and it's like society's only
forcin' you to go down one route.

My initial comment is presented as a question and is an attempt to open up debate
on the 'causes' of sexuality, which succeeds in encouraging other views (Glen's
social account and others follow). It is also a rejection of the biological deter-
minist view embodied by Sam's remarks and echoed in my further comment.
Asking critical questions like this can clearly be useful for provoking debate and
for helping the researcher feel as if she or he has challenged views perceived to be
narrow-minded or dangerous. It could also represent another exercise in power
assertion by ensuring that the researcher's perspective is heard. There is a delicate
balance for researchers to negotiate between respecting participants' views and
making careful, critical and perhaps more personal contributions to the research
encounter. Willott (1998) also comments on the difficulties of challenging participants' statements on the one hand, and recognising diverse, and at times
unpalatable, perspectives on the other.

> RV: 'Is this about an inability or refusal to resist challenging certain views,
> revealing my "social constructionist" leanings? Clearly, I am especially wary of
> claims about "nature", whether in research interviews, everyday conversation or
> media presentations, as repertoires of biological difference have been and
> continue to be used to "other" particular subjectivities. In relation to (straight) men
> and masculinities, it is often women and gay men who are subordinated. Sam's
> initial equation between "homosexuals" and "women's sexuality" reproduces

the conventional femininising of gay men, which I felt compelled to interrogate. I have known several gay men who patently subvert the effeminate stereotype and embody characteristics associated with conventional masculinities (toughness, detachment, physical strength etc.).'

Researcher as 'professional': defensively (mis)managing personal questions

The researcher rarely has it all his or her own way: control of the interaction does not inherently reside with the interviewer (Jorgenson, 1991). In some respects the interviewer is like a car salesperson, focused on the end result, instrumental, whilst the participant is the prospective buyer who is not necessarily committed to the purchase (Cicourel, 1964). There are moments during the research where roles are reversed and the researcher can experience a degree of vulnerability or self-consciousness:

Glen: It's quite interesting because we've all like talked about stuff and you just go 'Hmm, hmm' and 'I play football on Fridays' and 'I go for certain labels' [group laughter].
Interviewer: [lightly] So, what are you saying, Glen?
G: I'm saying we're all lowering our guard here and yours stays up!
I: What do you want me to talk about then? [laughter].
Jack: Do you think there's a difference between men working with other men and women because ...

I remember feeling anxious when Glen explicitly challenged my professional, detached stance ('What is the 'correct' procedure here?' I wondered). My response, as is evident, resorted to fending off Glen's advance with more questions for him, thus reverting to a detached role. Fortunately for me in this instance, I was 'saved' by another participant who conscientiously chose to explore the question of gender at work (arising from preceding talk).

RV: 'A very direct critique from Glen highlighting the manifest inequalities in relative contributions to the discussion – an exposé of my hitherto reticence to divulge my "self" beyond the confines of the "guarded" researcher-as-facilitator role. I was clearly unprepared for this, and felt like a bit of a "fraud". My subsequent evasiveness also strikes me as somehow unsatisfactory, and defensive, seeking to divert attention from myself to the others as quickly as possible. Perhaps I felt that disclosing personal *experiences* pertaining to masculine identities was inappropriate in a tutor–student context. After all, I would still have to teach these students and for them to know about, say, my drunken adventures or sexual fantasies, would be to risk public exposure within the university community, possibly compromising my professional position. So, although my detached veil was "seen through" by my students, and this provoked embarrassment for me, I suppose I felt this was the lesser of two evils.'

This instance raises questions about how to negotiate one's identity as a researcher during exchanges with participants – to what extent should the researcher exercise or relax 'self-discipline'? During one discussion I was asked: 'What I want to know is what the study is really about?' This was easier to handle because it didn't involve 'the personal' – an 'academic' response was appropriate. In another discussion, however, as well as asking for more clarification on the research ('How are you gonna analyse that?'), a personal view was most definitely sought – and on a 'difficult' subject. For example:

[The discussion had been about homosexuality]
Andy: What would you say about a person who wants anal sex with their partner?
Interviewer: I don't know, what do you think?
A: Well, I was asking you! [Group laughter]
I: I've no idea, it's open for debate.
A: Hmm, any comments on that Will?
Will: No, not really, I've never had that sort of feeling really.

Another example here of the researcher being taken by surprise, this time being explicitly requested to contribute a personal (rather than professional) opinion. Again, I made a rather feeble and transparent attempt to reflect the question back to the participant, who effectively recognises this ploy. My subsequent deflection, an appeal to other participants to take on this issue, is implicitly criticised by Andy ('Hmm') before he relieves me by redirecting the focus to another participant, Will.

> *RV:* 'I really didn't expect to be asked questions by the group – naively, perhaps. They were interested in gender issues and it is not surprising that they sought to include me in the discussions. My "I don't know" and (later) "I've no idea" denote uncertainty about how to respond and buy a little time for me to deflect the question back to the others. I also think that I had not really formed an opinion on the topic of anal sex – it was something outside my world. Feeling under pressure to provide a personal view, I opted for the safety of my researcher role. Is it another example too of me seeking to learn about (my) masculinity from the discourse of others? Apart from myself, it must have been an uncomfortable moment for some of the other group members like Andy, who steps in to take the debate in another direction.'

My responses to such enquires could be seen as disappointing in my steadfast maintenance of a neutral, questioning stance. What would other researchers have done? How does one manage 'the personal' in such a research setting? Are the participants manipulated or exploited (squeezed for data) by the researcher's avoidance (or a superficial impression) of active participation in the talk? Perhaps in a partial or unconscious attempt to address these issues, I invited the participants to reflect on the research during data collection:

Interviewer: Are you glad of this opportunity to talk?

Mal: The problem ... because *you're* not really opening up, recording material, you're sort of on the other side, I don't think you [participants] really open up.

I: I did think about having this in a pub [group laughter] but it would have been difficult to record. Obviously I want a situation which is as democratic as possible.

Glen: It's gettin' better though, isn't it? It was pretty tight, now it's more relaxed. We were a bit on edge, like we were being observed.

M: I'm not actually saying it's you!

I: I'm not taking it personally!

M: ... or what you stand for ... I think it's open, but I don't think it's the 'nitty gritty'.

G: It is pretty much though, isn't it? It isn't just all ... it's a bit more pushing in the opposite direction, bravado in the air, 'give her one' and all that, whereas here it's a bit more honest.

I think this strategy of encouraging participants to think critically and reflexively about the research in which they are participating is quite useful, in this case provoking an interesting debate about the 'authenticity' of accounts. Such discussions may highlight important participant perceptions of the researcher and of the research process and could provide suggestions about the format of future research. Again though, it places the focus on participant responses, with the researcher assuming a tacit or obscure presence – a point which Mal highlights (*'you're* not opening up, you're on the other side'). Perhaps researchers should think about this issue in advance, and try to decide how they will deal with personal questions – although, of course, some questions might well be unanticipated or tempt the researcher into potentially unhelpful self-disclosure. Ultimately, perhaps the best advice for researchers here is to enter interview situations with open minds, and to attempt some monitoring of self during and soon after the research encounter.

RV: 'I now consider these aspects of this study to be somewhat flawed. Certainly, I would do it differently in the future. It was one of my earliest forays into qualitative data collection and perhaps was not adequately thought through. These reflections may be seen as an attempt to rectify past mistakes. Yet, the data collected is very rich, and managing self-as-researcher is a complex affair regardless of degree of preparation or expertise. Am I letting myself off the hook?'

Final remarks

I have highlighted various dilemmas which qualitative researchers who attempt or imagine an unproblematically secure or conventional interview stance may well encounter whilst negotiating their position(s) during interview situations – dilemmas which centre on the management of the researcher's subjectivity. Admittedly, I had not fully discussed the format with the participants at the start of the research. A clear definition of roles agreed by all (e.g. the researcher signalling an (un)willingness to act as a co-participant) and increased participant involvement all round might go some way towards resolving researcher tensions over when and how much to remain 'in role'. Nonetheless, even if such consensus were established beforehand, the dynamics of the research situation might well prompt various players into resisting and reworking roles at given moments in the research process. Discourse analysts stress the notion of talk as emergent, dynamic, contradictory and negotiated (e.g. Potter & Wetherell, 1987). The question is how do we as researchers deal with our spontaneous and at times, perhaps, unwarranted personal interventions? This is not to advocate an attitude of professional detachment, but simply to encourage a critical examination of (often relevant and interesting) researcher subjectivity.

One response to this question is to reflect on a research encounter as soon as possible. If we could make notes immediately following a data collection event (which I didn't do in this project) then we could become sensitised to how we as researchers intervene at different points. We could then bear this in mind when next interacting with participants. Prior knowledge of the types of intervention we as researchers have made in previous research, as well as an openness to other potential reactions, will help us to contextualise and enrich the research analysis. Writing from a psychoanalytic perspective, Hollway and Jefferson (2000) advocate checking your impressions and interpretations with a colleague or co-researcher in order to identify potential unconscious identifications ('counter-transferences') and improve the quality of the analysis. For example, Hollway (in Hollway & Jefferson, 2000) provides an example where she noted mother–daughter transference and counter-transference during an interview with 'Jane'. This was evidenced by Jane telling her of experiences which only her mother knew about, and by Hollway dealing with Jane's children (who were present during the interview) in a (grand)motherly way, and by Jane associating her mother's view with Hollway's (unprompted) maternal advice about relationships.

Getting in touch with unwitting or unconscious researcher interventions in this way helps guard against presuming a fixed set of personal and intellectual positions consciously worked out in advance of data collection. For example, you may convince yourself that you're adopting an anti-sexist position yet your research could operate as an unconscious means of projecting your own prejudice on to 'legitimate' vulnerable targets! Rigorous reflections can help situate the research and highlight how data are co-produced, in this case with the help of considering unconscious intersubjective dynamics. Hollway and Jefferson (2000) also recommend second interviews with participants as a means of following up initial hypotheses and seeking deeper knowledge in a context where researcher and researched already know each other.

Summary

To conclude, qualitative researchers must resist the complacent assumption that research is informed by a clear set of definable personal and professional values. Careful scrutiny of research texts may well reveal evidence of other assumptions and practices which depart from well-considered positions and plans. The above analysis highlights several unanticipated roles adopted by this researcher within one study. It suggests that reflexive practice should recognise variability in researcher interventions and that the distinct functions served by specific contributions should be analysed. Although the retrospective analysis of interview transcripts carried out here is valuable for contextualising the research, *constant* reflection and revision of one's words and actions is imperative as data collection proceeds so that awareness and understanding of multiple researcher positions can be acquired. It is also suggested that qualitative researchers operating within a psychoanalytic tradition (e.g. Hollway & Jefferson, 2000) offer helpful advice for accessing emotions and assumptions which might otherwise remain repressed during data analysis and write-up. Clearly, reflexive practice does present many challenges for the qualitative researcher, but engaging with these can produce valuable insights into the production of researcher subjectivities and the management of the research process itself.

References

Ballinger, C. & Payne, S. (2000) Falling from grace or into expert hands? Alternative accounts about falling in older people. *British Journal of Occupational Therapy*, **63**, 573–9.

Burman, E. & Parker, I. (1993) *Discourse Analytic Research. Repertoires and Readings of Text in Action*. Routledge, London.

Circourel, A. (1964) *Method and Measurement in Sociology*. Free Press, New York.

Denzin, N. (2001) The reflexive interview and a performative social science. *Qualitative Research*, **1**(1), 23–46.

Gill, R. (1993) Justifying injustice: broadcaster's accounts of inequality. In *Discourse Analytic Research: Repertoires and Readings of Texts in Action* (Burman, E. & Parker, I., eds). Routledge, London.

Gough, B. (1998) Men and the discursive reproduction of sexism: repertoires of difference and equality. *Feminism & Psychology*, 8(1), 25–49.

Gough, B. (1999) 'Subject positions within discourse analysis: some reflexive dilemmas'. Paper given at *International Human Science Research Conference*, Sheffield Hallam University, July.

Gough, B. (in press) Psychoanalysis as resource for understanding emotional ruptures in the text: the case of defensive masculinities. *British Journal of Social Psychology*.

Gough, B. & Edwards, G. (1998) The beer talking: four lads, a carry out and the reproduction of masculinities. *The Sociological Review*, 46(3), 409–35.

Hollway, W. & Jefferson, T. (2000) *Doing Qualitative Research Differently: Free Association, Narrative and the Interview Method*. Sage Publications, London.

Jorgenson, J. (1991) Co-constructing the interviewer/ co-constructing 'family'. In *Research and Reflexivity* (Steier, F., ed.). Sage Publications, London.

Parker, I. (1994) Discourse analysis. In *Qualitative Methods in Psychology: A Research Guide* (Banister, P., Burman, E., Parker, I., Taylor, M. & Tindall, C., eds). Open University Press, Buckingham.

Potter, J. & Wetherell, M. (1987) *Discourse & Social Psychology: Beyond Attitudes and Behaviour*. Sage Publications, London.

Raphael-Reed, L. (1999) Troubling boys and disturbing discourses on masculinity and schooling: a feminist exploration of current debates and interventions concerning boys in school. *Gender and Education*, 11, 93–110.

Seale, C. (1999) *The Quality of Qualitative Research*. Sage Publications, London.

Skelton, C. (1998) Feminism and research into masculinities and schooling. *Gender & Education*, 10, 217–27.

Smith, J.A. (1995) Semi-structured interviewing and qualitative analysis. In *Rethinking Methods in Psychology* (Smith, J.A., Harré, R. & Van Langenhove, L., eds). Sage Publications, London.

Stainton-Rogers, R., Stenner, P., Gleeson, K. & Stainton-Rogers, W. (1995) *Social Psychology: A Critical Agenda*. Polity Press, Cambridge.

Steier, F. (1991) *Research and Reflexivity*. Sage Publications, London.

Taylor, C. & White, S. (2000) *Practising Reflexivity in Health and Welfare*. Open University Press, Buckingham.

Wetherell, M. & Edley, N. (1999) Negotiating hegemonic masculinity: imaginary positions and psycho-discursive practices. *Feminism & Psychology*, 9(3), 335–57.

Willott, S. (1998) An outsider within: a feminist doing research with men. In *Standpoints and Differences* (Henwood, K., Griffin, C. & Phoenix, A., eds). Sage Publications, London.

Willott, S. & Griffin, C. (1997) 'Wham, Bam, Am I a Man'? Unemployed men talk about masculinities. *Feminism & Psychology*, 7(1), 107–28.

PART IV

Reflexivity Through Collaboration

Qualitative research is rarely a solitary endeavour – It usually involves interacting with research participants, and often with other personnel, such as institutional 'gatekeepers' and academic colleagues. For some qualitative researchers, participant reflexivity should be recognised and exploited in order to facilitate an open and democratic research experience for all concerned. Clearly, this mode of research helps to challenge conventional roles and boundaries associated with research practice. As such, opportunities for reflexivity abound, such as sharing one's research questions and/or data analysis so that comments can be received and taken into account in subsequent drafts. Further, the researcher can help foster reflexivity on the part of co-researchers, say by asking them to reflect on their previous comments. But this giving up of research authority and 'expertise' can induce anxieties and tensions for researchers, and indeed for participants, who are at some level still wedded to traditional research roles. In Part IV, the challenge of working reflexively with others in different research contexts is explored.

Chapter 12 by Arvay articulates an innovative 'collaborative narrative approach' to qualitative research. Here, participants are asked to conduct their own analyses of the interview data and then to meet with the researcher to compare interpretations. A complex negotiated account is then produced, which the researcher then reflexively interrogates in order to identify her positions within the text and, ultimately, to produce what she feels to be the participant's story. Some of the power, benefits and difficulties experienced with this approach are highlighted. In a similar vein, Chapter 13 by Smith emphasises participant reflexivity. With reference to a research project on the transition to motherhood in which the women were interviewed at different time points, he shows how participants – and researcher – reach new understandings through discussing data previously collected. Reflexivity is thus enabled by the research design, and some interesting data are presented to illustrate the shifts and tensions pertaining to perceived meanings and identities throughout the research process. In Chapter 14 by Rowe, there is a discussion of a novel and distinctive approach to research where the researcher is also a participant. Drawing upon his experience of 'playback theatre', a form of improvised drama where members of the audience see their own stories played out on stage, he argues for and illustrates a reflexive methodology which addresses the tensions between the researcher maintaining critical distance from and becoming immersed in the phenomenon. An approach to research which embodies aspects of playback theatre, he argues, helps to vivify participants' accounts and shows how spontaneous engagement with the research process can have a powerful impact.

In contrast, Chapter 15 by McFadden and McCamley perceptively attends to some of the difficulties that researchers can be confronted with when working as part of a complex research matrix. For example, lack of clarity and disagreements about roles and responsibilities are reported with reference to their fascinating action research project on young people and sexual health. Reflexive practices such as maintaining research diaries and revisiting persistent issues with other researchers and participants are considered invaluable for promoting better quality research – from both researcher and participant perspectives. Chapter 16 by Barry also identifies how various reflexive strategies can be productively employed by a group of researchers. Reflecting on her experience while engaged on an exciting multidisciplinary project on doctor–patient communication, she discusses how the sharing of individually produced reflexive material within the team helps to render personal and academic agendas transparent. It is argued that such reflexive activities can improve both the functioning of the team and the quality of research.

CHAPTER 12

Doing reflexivity: a collaborative narrative approach

Marla J. Arvay

Positioning the self: author's story

I started my academic career doing quantitative research and always felt regret about not having expressed in my findings what I really wanted to know about my research questions. It was by accident that I stumbled upon qualitative research methods during my doctoral programme in counselling psychology. Attached to a survey on secondary traumatic stress were handwritten letters by participants expressing their heartfelt responses to the research questions. These letters and notes were moving and compelling. They contained the heart of the research aims that I had been striving to understand. I decided that I needed to find a way to do research that embodied the voices of my participants. After exploring various qualitative methodologies, I decided that I would have to fashion my own method – a *collaborative narrative method*. My aim with this method was to be collaborative, to attend to power relations within research and to deal with issues around voice and representation.

This method can be challenging. It is extensive, time-consuming and very personal. Collaborative research relationships are often fraught with power issues that can be difficult to sort through. In my approach, being reflexive means exploring how my personal experiences shape my understandings of my co-investigators and how viewing issues from multiple viewpoints affects our understandings of the phenomenon under study. It is about the ability to negotiate multiple and shifting meanings and for both parties to be able to voice their understandings equitably. My hope is to co-create research environments that are participatory and emancipatory.

Since my dissertation, I have been teaching qualitative research methods in the graduate programme in counselling psychology at the University of British Columbia. A very large part of the curriculum is devoted to issues of reflexivity in terms of relations of power in research, researcher subjectivity, the interpretive process and representation in research texts. As a counselling psychologist I am also able to bring the reflexive lessons learned through collaborative, narrative research initiatives to my work as a narrative therapist. Narrative inquiry has influenced my understanding of my experiences as a narrative therapist – how reality is co-constructed, dialogical, relational, contextual and partial. Narrative inquiry as an epistemology has bridged my understanding of others and self into both my professional and personal life.

Introduction

The focus of this chapter is to offer an illustration of reflexive human and social science research using a collaborative narrative method. The collaborative narrative method (Arvay, 1998, 2002) was developed during my doctoral research while investigating the experience of secondary traumatic stress among female trauma psychotherapists. This method is located within narrative inquiry (Mishler, 1986; Polkinghorne, 1988; Riessman, 1993), a methodology rooted in social constructionist and post-structuralist epistemologies. Narrative inquiry differs from other forms of research due to its focus on the dialogical nature of knowledge and its emphasis on the social world as a site where power relations are played out. Meanings are always disputable depending upon who is speaking to whom and the power relations either held or perceived to be held within these interactions. As a relatively new methodology, narrative inquiry attempts to demonstrate the co-constructed nature of knowledge produced through human and social science research. Acknowledging that multiple perspectives influence knowledge production, narrative researchers are plagued with questions concerning re-presentation and voice in the research text and the difficulties of interpretation. All of these concerns are fundamentally about reflexivity. Reflexivity from a narrative perspective scrutinises the researcher's process and examines how power relations are attended to both within the research relationship and in the construction of the research narratives. Reflexivity is demonstrated in this chapter through the collaborative research relationships and in-depth interpretive processes of analyses described.

The *collaborative narrative method* (Arvay, 1998, 2002) is a reflexive qualitative method involving seven stages within the research process:

(1) Setting the stage
(2) The performance: co-constructing the research interview
(3) The transcription process
(4) Four collaborative interpretive readings
(5) The interpretive interview
(6) Writing the narratives
(7) Sharing the story

Stage one: setting the stage – a reflexive preliminary interview

To begin the research process, it is important to meet with all the co-investigators (participants) to engage in a pre-interview conversation and to facilitate contemplation about the research process. Unlike action research where the participants and researchers determine the aims of the research together, in this method the research questions and focus of research are predetermined by the researcher. However, this first stage of the method could be modified to be more participatory and emancipatory from the start by following action research models in the selection and recruitment of participants.

The main purposes of the preliminary interview are:

- To develop rapport.
- To begin facilitating a dialogue pertaining to the research question.
- To explain the research process by detailing all the stages of the research.
- To describe the roles and responsibilities that both the co-investigator and the researcher will have in the research.
- To articulate one's own values regarding the research relationship.
- To explain the basic philosophical values upon which the research design rests (e.g. the storied nature of our lives; that the self is constituted through the stories we tell; that telling our stories can be a transformative experience; that stories always change with each retelling; and that the researcher can never hope to recapture the lived moment of the telling in the research text).

Taking time at this phase of the research to inform the co-investigators about the nature of their participation and to lay the groundwork for the research relationship will prove invaluable later during the interpretive phase of the research. I usually share the reasons why I am interested in the research topic with the co-investigators before we start the process. As a note of caution, participants could well drop out of the study at this point because they recognise the demanding investment of their time.

Once the stage has been set, the researcher must evaluate whether the potential co-investigator has the time, interest and energy for this lengthy research method. After articulating the research goals, the research process and the lengthy time commitment, the co-investigator determines whether informed consent can be given.

Stage two: the performance

Understanding the research interview as 'joint action' (Shotter, 1999), I am always conscious of the role that I am playing in the construction of the 'script'. Using a model of collaborative research explicated by Ellis *et al.* (1997), my goal is to 'invite stories' (Polanyi, 1985) from my co-investigators concerning their experience with the research question. Although this 'inviting' may sound simple, it is actually a very complex act because it requires more than interviewing skills. The ease of inviting stories pertains to the everyday act of engaging in conversation and the difficulty of inviting stories has to do with the level of attunement or reflexivity involved in the act of co-constructing the research narrative. It is about entering what John Shotter (1999) refers to as the 'third space' by being present to it and trusting that the process will unfold – a leap of faith that meaning-making activities will develop dialogically. The narrative researcher takes up a dual consciousness – performing the story as narrator and reflecting on the story being told as researcher, continually moving between these and other subjectivities as the conversation unfolds.

I envision research participants as co-investigators and co-actors in this research performance, not as respondents answering upon request, nor as informants merely imparting information. As a performance, the conversation is complex on many levels. Both the co-investigator and the researcher hold multiple 'I' positions in the exchange as our various possible selves interact (Hermans *et al.*, 1993). I am also aware that inviting a co-investigator's story is more than just opening up the conversation or asking 'good' questions. It entails attending to the narrative account at both the micro-level of the individual experience of the narrator, and at the macro-level of cultural discourse. It means being engaged at both an experiential level and a reflexive level – again, it is about holding dual consciousness. I ask the co-investigator about the paradoxes, the silences and pauses in their stories and invite the co-investigator to respond to me in the same manner. We attempt to uncover the contradictions and to articulate tacit knowledge through metaphor, body language and by comparing similar experiences.

Self-disclosure concerning the personal experiences of the researcher often initiates authentic dialogue and opens up an opportunity for the researcher to re-examine her or his own interpretations or beliefs. There were several instances during a recent research project on secondary trauma where I offered an anecdote, shared my feelings about my co-investigator's experience, or told a parallel story. As an example, when one of my co-investigators stated that she started seeing perpetrators everywhere and knew she was acting irrationally, I shared with her one of my experiences working with sexually abused children. As I became more aware of the risks to children, I began seeing potential paedophiles everywhere. We mutually explored the meanings of our shared experiences. We laughed and cried together, and struggled to understand what it all meant. On one occasion, I was challenged to come down from my researcher's perch when my co-investigator asked what I meant when I said, 'Oh, that's interesting!' Embarrassed by my 'power-over' comment, I explained that I had momentarily slipped away into trauma theory as her previous comment had resonated with the findings of a research article I had read that morning.

A reflexive, collaborative interview could entail at least a three- to four-hour session. At the completion of the interview, I ask the co-investigator to write down any thoughts he or she might have about the interview process as I engage in writing field notes. If the co-investigator does not have the time to complete this task, I write these process notes immediately after the session in private. For example, in the above scenario, I wrote down my feelings and insights into being dethroned from the research perch.

Stage three: the transcription process

Transcription as an interpretive practice underscores the researcher's theoretical and epistemological assumptions about research (Kvale, 1996; Denzin, 1997; Richardson, 1997). The method of transcription for this narrative method employs models of transcription described by Susan Chase (1995) and Catherine Kohler Riessman (1993). I preface the description of my transcription procedures with two caveats. First, I recognise that the exact reproduction of the speech act is impossible. All we can do is attempt to reproduce the communicative events as closely as possible – they will never be exact (Denzin, 1997; Richardson, 1997). Second, we cannot reproduce past events. Our stories (and the record of these stories) do not mirror the world as lived because our stories are constructed retrospectively and, in this research method, they are co-constructed perfor mances. As an analogy, there are qualitative and interpretive differences between writing a play, being an actor in a play, watching the play, or reading the play.

The co-investigators' audiotapes are transcribed twice. The first transcription is produced as a *rough draft*. Carefully listening to the speech events, I record each aspect of the speech produced (e.g. laughter, pauses, silences and gaps, hedging, crying, tone of voice) and also note any aspect of the speech act that is not audible on the audiotape, but is recorded in written form in my field notes (e.g. body language, movement, facial expressions, positioning, environmental influences and other contextual cues). For instance, one field note in the secondary trauma study observed the happy, smiling countenance of the interviewee, yet her actual words were shocking and violent as she described her response to one of her clients' trauma experiences. Her body language contradicted her oral speech. I was able to go back later and ask about this paradox. In narrative inquiry, it is important to attend to the storying process (how the story is told) as much as the content of the story. It is in the *construction of the narrative* that selves are positioned, constituted and contextualised.

For the second draft, I follow a listening method developed by James Gee (1986, 1991) as described in Catherine Kohler Riessman's (1993) text on narrative analysis. I re-transcribe the conversation by displaying the text of the rough draft in *stanza form*, where each episode of the narrative is kept together in a series of lines and the tone of speech and pace are marked. Each episode that is conceptualised as a story within the larger narrative is marked at its beginning and ending by double spacing. A bold font is used to indicate emphasis in the speaker's tone of voice, followed by a bracketed word indicating the actual tone of voice used. Italics are used to emphasise emotional expression followed by a bracketed word indicating my interpretation and/or level of the emotion. Both speakers are included in the transcript and when speech overlaps, the researcher's speech is bracketed with '{}' to show that it has been spoken simultaneously with the co-investigator. All hesitations and pauses are written into the text by using three ellipsis points. I pay close attention to the pauses in the text during the interpretation stage of this model. Pauses and hesitations may be text markers that point to places in the conversation where tacit knowledge is at work. Here is an example of the transcription practice using Gee's (1991) stanza form.

Co-investigator:
It was at this cloistered college
That my world view
About good and evil
Started to get shaken up ...   Pause 3 seconds; voice quiet/low

An old childhood friend
Confided to me
On a visit one weekend
In my first year
That she had been sexually assaulted
By her uncle and cousins
Throughout her childhood.

I didn't overreact ...   Pause 5 seconds
I just listened and tried to comfort her.

I seemed to have an intuitive sense
About hearing this story ...   Pause 3 seconds
Where this comes from
I don't know (laughs lightly)   Field note: I think she does know; ask
                                                her later.

Later that year ...

The last transcription task, before entering into the analysis of the narrative, is to identify *narrative episodes*: places in the text where stories begin and conclude or are taken up again later, that is, 'listening for entrance and exit talk' (Riessman, 1993, p.13). I attempt to identify stories within stories in order to understand the temporal sequencing of the storyline and to determine the unfolding of the plot.

I'd like to emphasise that transcription is an *interpretive process* that is always partial – in any specified notation system, some aspects of speech are included while others are excluded (Mishler, 1986). The inclusion/exclusion dimension of transcription practices only points to the assumptions held by the transcriber or interpreter (Richardson, 1990; Kvale, 1996; Denzin, 1997; Ellis *et al.*, 1997). As a reflexive practice, it is important for the researcher to scrutinise his/her own transcription practices in order to uncover assumptions about what is an important speech act and what is not, and more importantly, why.

Stage four: four collaborative interpretive readings of the transcript

In this stage of the research process, the co-investigators and I collaboratively participate to engage the transcribed text in a meaningful way. I prepare a reading guide for my co-investigators to follow. I photocopy the transcript onto 11 × 17-inch paper and draw four columns in the right margin. The co-investigators are given four different coloured pens and asked to interpret their own transcript during *four separate readings*. The general instructions are as follows.

'The following is a guide to assist you in interpreting the text. This process entails at least four readings of the text and perhaps more as the research process unfolds. I am asking you to be the interpreter of your own transcript. The purpose of each reading is to approach the text from a different standpoint ... If there are other readings that you would like to engage in, please call me in order that I may do the same so that our interpretive processes coincide.'

Reading for content

In the first reading, I ask the co-investigators to read the transcription for coherence concerning the content of the research interview. I ask them to make changes if they feel that the text needs to be clearer or expanded upon and to make corrections if they find errors in this first read through.

Reading for the self of the narrator

In the second reading, I ask the co-investigators to read for the narrator's self: 'Read for the narrator's various "I" positions. Who is telling this story? How is she situated in this story? What is she feeling? What are her struggles? How does she present herself? What meaning is she trying to convey? What parts of self does she share and what parts are kept hidden? Why? As the protagonist of her own tale, what does she want to convey to the reader?' The purpose of this reading is to bring to light the ways in which the narrator constructs herself in the text. The co-investigator steps out of her or his previous role as participant and steps into a new role as interpreter of the research text. This is another example of the collaborative narrative method as a reflexive practice – the co-investigator reflects on her own narration and ponders on the self that is constructed through a dialogical research method (Hoskins & Arvay, 1999).

Reading for the research question

In the third reading, I ask the co-investigators to read for their response to the research question. For example, in a study on secondary traumatic stress among trauma counsellors (Arvay, 1998), I asked the co-investigators to find places in the text where they articulated their struggle with secondary traumatic stress. 'What meaning does the narrator make of this struggle? How does she make sense out of her experiences? What is "not said", or implied? What are the contradictions between her words and actions and/or your interpretations as the reader? What metaphors does she use and how do they help in making meaning? Take time to reflect on this reading. Perhaps there will be places in the text that resonate with you but you may not be able to articulate what it is – make note of these places for our discussion later.'

In this reading, I am looking for the details of their personal experience with the research question, but I am also looking for layers of tacit knowledge. I focus on those places in the text (including my research notes from the interview) where the co-investigators have disrupted the flow of conversation – places where they took a moment to pause or 'arrest' – in which there appeared to be a shift in consciousness. Shotter (1999) refers to these as 'striking', 'moving', or 'arresting' moments, as moments that have the possibility to 'originate new forms of life in us' (p. 7). This interpretive reading process is 'reflexivity-in-action'. It requires an attunement with the research text and involves multiple layering of meaning-making as the reader moves from the 'story-as-told' to other possible inter-pretations of the meanings constructed in narrating lived experience. The story is never finished. Our research narratives are always changing through dialogue either in conversations with others or in conversations with self.

Reading for relations of power and culture

The final reading in this collaborative narrative method is a critical one. The instructions in this phase are along these lines: 'As you read the text, look for suggestions of power or gender imbalances. In what ways does the narrator struggle with issues regarding inequities? Where is she or he silenced? When does he or she lose his or her voice? Is the narrator conscious of the power or political influences in her or his life or of the influences of culture? How do you understand his or her history/context/social world? In what ways are her or his "personal realities" challenged?' In this reading, I am attempting to articulate with the co-investigator the cultural discourse at work in the text. The level of reflexivity in this reading emphasises a broader scope, a cultural critique of the forces (i.e. political, social, psychological, biological, technical etc.) that are at work in the construction of self narrated in the research text.

Interpreting the self of the researcher in the transcript

As the co-investigators complete these four interpretive readings, I also interpret their transcriptions using these four reading guidelines. However, I also apply the four interpretive readings to my *own* interactions in the transcript. Believing that the research interview is a co-construction, it is imperative to know the ways in which I, as the researcher, influence the production of the research transcript. Steier (1991) defines reflexivity as a turning back on one's experiences upon oneself wherein the self to which this bending back refers is predicated and must also be understood as socially constructed. He states that 'this folding back may unfold as a spiraling, if we allow for multiple perspectives, and acknowledge that the same self may be different as a result of its own self-pointing' (Steier, 1991, p. 3). I re-read the transcript four times applying the reading guide to myself and make notes in the margins in a different colour from the co-investigators'. These notes were crucial to my final interpretation and writing of their narrative accounts.

Stage five: the interpretive interview – a collaborative interpretation of the text

In the next conversation with the co-investigators, we retrospectively, collaboratively and reflexively discuss the interpretations from the four readings, then listen and respond to each other's renderings. The discussion typically lasts two to three hours in length and should be audiotaped. From my experience, this conversation is usually very moving and informative as we explore the meanings of the metaphors, make attempts to comprehend ambiguous parts of the narrative account, and struggle to see the cultural implications of our interpretations. Some of the questions at this stage are: 'What do you think this means? Where do you think you learned that? What were your feelings about that? There seems to be something left out here – something not said. What do you think this section is about? What do you wish could have happened? What did you learn from this experience? There is something that I see in this section, what do you think? How does my interpretation fit with yours?' And finally, I ask, 'Is there anything more you would like to add to this interpretation?' Remembering that this was an interactive, dialogical co-construction, I also apply these questions to my *own* participation and interpretations. I share these with the co-investigators and record my responses in a journal to assist me in writing their stories. The interpretive interview is best done one-to-one due to the complexity of the process; however, a group interpretive interview may be possible

Stage six: writing stories

The next task before writing the research narratives is to summarise our interpretive readings into one blended text. I first develop clarity on each of the readings, and then devise a plot line placing the episodes in sequential and temporal order. I typically write the stories as first person accounts – a literary device aiming to bring their stories 'back to life'. These narrative accounts are a joint construction, carefully crafted through a reflexive and collaborative research process. Unlike traditional psychological research that objectifies participants' lives by writing their findings in the third person and by reducing their participants' stories to categorical classification or short quotes, this method resists such reductionistic tendencies and makes every attempt to fashion a tale that is embodied – a tale that is coherent, compelling and revealing of the storyteller's intentions. Although researchers conducting narrative analyses can also be criticised for engaging in reductionistic practices, this particular method attempts to expand on the story as told to include the researcher's perspectives while weaving into the text the collaborative analyses produced through the four interpretive readings. The narrative is written as a story-in-progress. The co-investigator now becomes *co-editor* and has the final word on the form and the content of the narrative account. The form of the narrative account could be a story, a poem, a play or an autobiography, to name a few.

Acknowledging that there is no final version, the authors (researcher and co-investigator) negotiate some of the interpretations made possible through the interpretive readings. The narrative accounts produced using this method often do not resemble 'modernist tales' with a clear plot line, building to a crisis point and ending with a resolution. Often they become 'postmodern tales' with issues left unresolved, in a chaotic entanglement for the reader to sort through. These forms of narrative representation often contain contradictions and ambiguity – like 'real' life, a life in progress, a chapter not yet finished.

You, as the reader, may be overwhelmed at this point by the time constraints involved in this collaborative narrative method. If you don't have the luxury of this kind of time, you could do the narrative method utilising the four readings without the collaborative element. However, I believe the interpretive process will be compromised. The narratives without the collaborative process become the *researcher's* stories and rely solely on the researcher's interpretation of the meaning of the co-investigators' lived experiences. Collaboration throughout the research process, particularly the analyses of the transcript, enhances participatory, and perhaps, emancipatory human science research.

Stage seven: sharing the story

In this final section I now move away from 'telling' you, the reader, about reflexive research and into 'showing' a small portion of a recent study using this narrative method. I want to share a story about the process of interpreting the 'other' and the emotional struggle that ensued upon completion of this research project. My story highlights the complexity of doing reflexive research and the difficult challenge for human science researchers in the task of writing the 'other' into being. This story poses important questions concerning who has authority and authorship over the research texts we produce. It is also a story about redemption. It is a tale about lessons learned in doing reflexive research using this collaborative narrative method.

Taking the story back

As I drove through the small rural community outside the city limits, I wondered why I had not brought the directions that Donna had given me. I was driving into unknown territory – no landmarks, no map. I was anxious whether the story I had written about her life was too raw. As I drove into her driveway that sunny afternoon I wondered if Donna was ready to hear or read this version of those three hours spent analysing her transcript. I was concerned that she would have a negative reaction to the narrative that I had written about her life. Questions filled my head. What if she starts to cry? What if she gets angry with me? What will I do? How will I defend myself? I had taken her tormented moments, all of those deep sobs and heavy sighs, the disjointed speech of a distraught woman and reconstituted it into a research account. Not only had I fashioned a coherent tale, but I had also written in the first person, as if it were my story.

I had written Donna into being, given her a coherence that had not been present in the research interview or in the interpretive interview. I had filled in every heavy sigh with text, every tear with a metaphor, every disjointed phrase with purpose and clarity. I had also included in Donna's tale my own story, the researcher's perspective. I could reveal myself as author and interpreter through the character of the protagonist of this tale. Donna could speak for Donna and me. However, I could reside safely, privately, in the shadow of her story. Donna was exposed in the text, but I was not, which gave rise to these feelings of anxiety as I approached her home. I wondered whether Donna would remember the joint conversation in the interpretive interview process in which we analysed her story together, co-constructing meaning. Donna's story was really our story and now I was confronted with the overwhelming task of sharing it with her. What would she say?

I realised as I reached her driveway that I felt some angst because I had appropriated her voice, used her experience as a catalyst to fashion my own and had 'dressed-up' her messy text, her chaotic description, for the purpose of writing 'good science'. I wanted to write an embodied research text full of the emotionality present during its creation. However, I could not merely provide transcript data because it was not clear or complete. Donna's interview was lengthy and full of stops and starts. There were flashbacks to previous events interchanged with present events and in-the-moment awarenesses. Her story construction process was complicated and at times disjointed. The transcript did not capture the fullness of those three hours at my kitchen table where Donna had poured out her story because a transcript cannot bring to life to the reader the lived experience. I also had to incorporate the interpretive interview into the final research text, which moved the story as given into a whole new realm. Added to this was the interpretive interview that I had conducted upon myself as a co-narrator of the original transcript – I had written myself as co-narrator into the text. Since the process of writing Donna's story was complicated and multi-layered, I wondered if she would be able to understand the complexity of this reflexive research method. I was on a quest for absolution: what I really wanted was Donna's blessing and permission to tell the story.

I took the file folder off the passenger seat and got out of the car. I approached the front door and rang the bell. As I entered, she asked me if I cared for a cup of tea – I fell back on these words, remembering the last time we had travelled down this road together. 'Donna, would you like a cup of tea before you go?' 'Now would you like to hear the real story?' she replied. Recalling that moment, I asked myself what can of worms would be opened over this new cup of tea? I said, 'Yes', stalling, trying to get a sense of her mood. We finally settled at her dining room table and I opened the file folder. 'Well, here it is Donna. Do you want to read it yourself? Do you want a pencil to write over it as you read? Maybe you prefer to read the whole story first and then go back and make changes while we talk?' 'No', she said, 'Why don't you just read it to me while I listen and drink my tea?' I was struck by her words. How would I read it? She was asking me to perform the role of her, to take up her voice in her presence. I wanted to flee, to say, 'Thanks for the tea, but I've got to run.' Instead I said, 'Donna, I have used poetic licence to craft a tale that I hoped might capture the experience you shared with me. I tried to piece together all the threads and write a story that was compelling, emotional, and I hope realistic. I tried to write as if I had lived through that evening with you, Donna. So here it is. . . .'

Summary

Ruth Behar (1996) in her book, *The Vulnerable Observer,* writes 'If you don't mind going places without a [traditional] map, follow me' (1996, p.33). This collaborative narrative method is about going places without a traditional human science research map. It is about doing and writing research that involves researchers' critical reflections on issues of emotionality in research, positions of power and voice in research, and the dialogical nature of the research process. This narrative method holds promise as a dialogically embodied, collaboratively focused and reflexive process for doing human science research.

References

Arvay, M.J. (1998) *Secondary Traumatic Stress: Stories of Struggle and Hope.* PhD dissertation. University of Victoria, Victoria, BC, Canada.

Arvay, M.J. (2002) Putting the heart back into human science research. In *Studies in Meaning: Exploring Constructivist Psychology* (Raskin, J.D. & Bridges, S.K., eds). Pace University Press, New York.

Behar, R. (1996) *The Vulnerable Observer: Anthropology that Breaks your Heart.* Beacon, Boston.

Chase, S. (1995) Taking narrative seriously: consequences for method and theory in interview studies. In *Interpreting Experience: The Narrative Study of Lives* (Josselson, R. & Lieblich, A., eds). Sage Publications, Thousand Oaks, CA.

Denzin, N.K. (1997) *Interpretive Ethnography: Ethnographic Practices for the 21st Century.* Sage Publications, Thousand Oaks, CA.

Ellis, C., Kiesinger, C.E. & Tillmann-Healy, L.M. (1997) Interactive interviewing. In *Reflexivity and Voice.* (Hertz, R., ed.). Sage Publications, Thousand Oaks, CA.

Gee, J.P. (1986) Units in the production of narrative discourse. *Discourse Processes*, 9, 391 122.

Gee, J.P. (1991) A linguistic approach to narrative. *Journal of Narrative and Life History*, 1(1), 15–39.

Hermans, H.J.M., Rijks, T.I. & Kempen, H.J. (1993) Imaginal dialogues in the self: theory and method. *Journal of Personality*, 61(2), 207–36.

Hoskins, M. & Arvay, M.J. (1999) The quagmire of researching the self: implications for constructivism. *Constructivism in the Human Sciences*, 4(1), 13–31.

Kvale, S. (1996) *InterViews: An Introduction to Qualitative Research Interviewing.* Sage Publications, Thousand Oaks, CA.

Mishler, E.G. (1986) *Research Interviewing: Context and Narrative.* Harvard University Press, Cambridge, MA.

Polanyi, L. (1985) *Telling the American Story: A Structural and Cultural Analysis of Conversational Storytelling.* Ablex, Norwood, NJ.

Polkinghorne, D.E. (1988) *Narrative Knowing and the Human Sciences.* State University of New York Press, Albany, NY.

Richardson, L. (1990) *Writing Strategies: Researching Diverse Audiences.* Sage Publications, Newbury Park, CA.

Richardson, L. (1997) *Fields of Play: Constructing an Academic Life.* Rutgers University Press, New Brunswick, NJ.

Riessman, C.K. (1993) *Narrative Analysis.* Sage Publications, Newbury Park, CA.

Shotter, J. (1999) 'Dialogue, depth, and life inside responsive orders: from external observation to participatory understanding'. Paper presented at conference on *Dialogues on Performing Knowledge*, Stockholm, Sweden.

Steier, F. (ed.) (1991) *Research and Reflexivity.* Sage Publications, Newbury Park, CA.

CHAPTER 13

Shifting identities: the negotiation of meanings between texts and between persons

Jonathan A. Smith

Positioning the self: author's story

I completed my PhD in 1990 and since then have been an academic psychologist, first at Keele University, then at the University of Sheffield and now at Birkbeck, University of London. I have articulated a particular qualitative approach, interpretative phenomenological analysis (IPA; Smith, 2003), and applied it to issues primarily in the social psychology of health. IPA is broadly phenomenological in its concern with understanding how participants make sense of their experiences but it also recognises the important role for the researcher in that process. IPA represents a *double hermeneutic* in which the researcher tries to make sense of the participant trying to make sense of their experience.

I see reflexivity as central to the human project, as people reflect on themselves, their activities, and what is happening around them. This process is both constitutive and constructive as the process of reflection can lead to one of change. I think George Herbert Mead has made the greatest contribution to thinking in this area. As indicated above, it can also be argued that the researcher is involved in a parallel process of reflection, so that one way to describe the meeting of researcher and participant in the research project itself is as a 'dialogical reflexivity'.

Introduction

In this chapter I will argue that reflexivity is a central feature of understanding the nature of the person in psychology. The form of reflexivity presented is derived from George Herbert Mead (1934). The chapter also argues for the close conjunction of theoretical positions and methodological practices. It presents a set of methodological practices specifically intended to facilitate the realisation of aspects of the reflexive thesis outlined and illustrative examples are provided of these practices. I start with an exploration of the theory and then move on to describe its relevance within a research project. I see the challenge as realising empirically the theoretical propositions about reflexivity offered by Mead and others.

Self as reflexive being

Mead saw the person as a socially constructed but reflexive and, therefore, potentially agentic being. Mead described himself as a social behaviourist and this prepares us for his radical social constructionism – the social rather than biological fashioning of the individual, society and culture preceding identity or 'personhood'. Mead was not an anti-mentalist however. He argued that although the self initially arose from social interaction, the individual develops through the internal, symbolic replay of the social nexus:

> 'After a self has arisen, it in a certain sense provides for itself its social experiences, and so we can conceive of an absolutely solitary self . . . who still has himself [*sic*] as a companion, and is able to think and to converse with himself as he had communicated with others' (1934, p.140).

Thus, reflexivity is central to Mead's notion of the person for, while mind is primarily a social construct, 'there is nothing odd about a product of a given process contributing to, or becoming an essential factor in the further development of that process' (1934, p.226).

Writing in 1980, Gergen echoes this strand of Mead:

> 'In each case the individual may turn to review his or her patterns of thought or feeling with the effect of alteration. And it is argued any internal tendency, habit, association or feeling may be critically confronted by the individual and the result may be self-generated modification or alteration. The internal system may thus continue to operate in itself without benefit from environmental inputs, and may undergo autonomous internally generated transformation' (p.39).

In a useful discussion of Mead, Burkitt (1991) points to the number of dualisms he confronted and deconstructed: self/society; mind/behaviour; structure/agency. This last pair is especially pertinent to current debate as it indicates that social construction does not necessarily signify social determinism. This is a point taken up in, for example, Butler's (1990) conception of a liberationary form of post-structuralist feminism:

> 'Paradoxically the reconceptualization of identity as an effect that is produced or generated opens up possibilities of agency that are insidiously foreclosed by positions that take identity categories as foundational and fixed. For an identity to be an effect means that it is neither fatally determined nor fully artificial and arbitrary' (p.147).

For Butler, the task for feminism is 'to affirm the local possibilities of intervention through participating in precisely those practices of repetition that constitute identity and therefore present the immanent possibility of contesting them' (1990, p.147).

Reflexivity then, offers us a model of person which is not determinatively fixed, whether by essence or by discourse. According to the reflexive thesis, the material of identity is initially derived from the culture and discourse in which the individual is situated. This material is then fashioned by that individual alone, or working dynamically with others, in order to construct and reconstruct an identity.

This model of a person has implications for the status of the accounts people provide of themselves. Such accounts provide access to identities not because they transparently or semi-transparently reveal an inner core or essence but because identities are the very accounts and stories people tell themselves and others – whether orally, in writing, or sub-vocally in their heads. Giddens (1991) captures a component of this quite nicely:

> 'Self-identity is not a distinctive trait, or even a collection of traits possessed by the individual. It is the self as reflexively understood by the person in terms of her or his biography. Identity here still presumes continuity across time and space: but self-identity is such continuity as interpreted reflexively by the agent ... A person's identity is not to be found in behaviour nor, important though this is, in the reactions of others but in the capacity to keep a particular narrative going' (pp.53–4).

Giddens' position has been taken up by a number of social scientists, e.g. Pavis *et al.* (1998); Denscombe (2001). This position distinguishes a reflexive theory of person or identity from an essentialist one. What relation does it have to a more discursively oriented position? It suggests that accounts from participants provide more than illustrations of linguistically determined and locally contingent accounting procedures. Rather, by telling their stories, people are simultaneously revealing their identities and fulfilling certain socially sanctioned discursive roles. The thesis seems to have implications for agency. People's accounts represent particular narratives which have been fashioned from, but fashioned uniquely from, the social discourses in which they are situated. These are narratives, then, for which people can be held responsible, that are authorial and accountable.

This reflexive thesis also has implications for the 'realistic' status of life stories, biographies or autobiographies alluded to earlier. If the focus of one's research is on the effect of events, meetings and interactions on people, and if personal identities are constructed by individuals in the course of telling stories to themselves and others, then the real project lies in analysing those stories or accounts, not in attempting to discover the events of a real life. Indeed whether or not the event actually happened is not the point of such work for, as Thomas succinctly puts it, 'If men [*sic*] define situations as real, they are real in their consequences' (quoted in Allport, 1947, p.22). So accounts obtained from respondents in the course of conducting research projects should be analysed as pieces of identity, and should be considered, at least primarily, as 'documents *of* life' (Plummer, 2001) rather than as documents *about* life.

The reflexive self and biographical reconstruction

One domain where reflexivity is foregrounded is in biography or autobiography where an individual is reflecting on how the self has developed over time. Of course the particular twist offered by the reflexive turn is to view the auto-biographical account as demonstrating how a story of the self is currently con-structed rather than seeing the account as a veridical record of the person's history. This turn is reflected in some conceptions of life-span developmental psychology. For example, Datan *et al.* (1987) suggest that adult personality or life-span psychology should be concerned more with how the individual creates a sense of order or biography rather than assuming or measuring the order itself.

This turn to a reflexive self, and the study of order as constructed rather than given, also suggests a dynamic role for memory in the process of constructing identity:

> 'All I wish to propose is that for all practical purposes the past exists only when we re-create it by training our thinking on it, or that the past as individual and collective history cannot be recovered but has to be recon-structed' (Wyatt, 1964, pp.315–19).

This reconstructive view of memory is in line with some models within main-stream experimental psychology (Gleitman, 1999) although such models are not generally concerned with relatively macro-psychological features such as bio-graphical organisation (Loftus' work on reconstructive processes in eyewitness testimony marks an exception, e.g. Manning & Loftus, 1996).

Faced with a biographical account, how does one determine self-constructive activity as envisaged by Datan *et al.* (1987)? Obviously one can speculate on constructive processes occurring and one can examine rhetorical devices being employed. However, at a more substantive level, it may prove difficult to dif-ferentiate, analytically, between a posited 'real' history unfolding and a personal story being constructed. Access to independent sources may also not resolve the issue because, following from arguments made earlier, much of what is inter-esting or important psychologically in a biography concerns subjective con-structs: how the person conceives a particular situation at a certain time point rather than supposedly objective events themselves. And no independent ver-ification of these personal constructs is obtainable.

The challenge, then, is to find ways of realising empirically the important theoretical propositions about reflexivity and self-construction offered by Giddens, Datan *et al.* and others, to design studies explicitly aimed at revealing self-constructive processes occurring in autobiography. One possibility is to compare accounts of an event produced in real time with later retrospective reports of the same time period. If an analysis reveals systematic differences between the accounts, this would strongly point to reflexive, reconstructive strategies employed by the participant. The argument would be that, in subsequent reflection on an event or stage in the past, the participant now reconstrues it. The important point is that such analysis enables empirical verification of the reflexive, constructive processes involved.

I have conducted a study using this type of design. In order to harness optimally the propensity for self-reflection or reflexivity, I worked with participants going through a major life transition: in this case the process of becoming a mother. I considered that I would be more likely to obtain detailed accounts which could be compared across time if I asked participants to reflect on events which were of particular significance to them. This study therefore followed a small number of women through their first pregnancy and compared their contemporaneous accounts of how the pregnancy was affecting them with retrospective accounts of the same time period, but written after the child was born.

I visited the women at three points during their pregnancy – at three, six and nine months – and asked them to consider how they felt about the pregnancy. Questions were posed so as to try to obtain an account of how the woman perceived pregnancy as affecting her sense of identity. Then, five months after the birth of the child, I asked each woman to write a retrospective account of the pregnancy. She was asked to think back to herself at the three relevant time points and write a short account of how she thought she was at that time. Equivalent cue terms to those in the real-time meetings were used. Each woman had no access to the accounts she had produced in real time.

I then compared the real-time and retrospective accounts for each woman. Many discrepancies were discovered and these point to a number of reconstructive narratives: the women were, through a process of personal reflexive engagement, retrospectively reconstructing a story of what their pregnancy was like. The reconstructions fall into three broad categories:

- Glossing over apparent difficulties; typically late pregnancy is perceived at the time as a time of anxiety whereas in retrospect there is some idealisation of this period.
- Construction of a progressive narrative through the transition, suggesting personal development and downplaying any decline.
- Establishing a sense of order and continuity through the transition, e.g. between the person who was pregnant and the person who is now a mother.

To illustrate how these reconstructions play out, one example of the first category is provided below. The complete study is reported in Smith (1994a). The names of participants and other people referred to by them have been changed throughout the chapter to protect confidentiality.

Clare was typical of the women in that she reported considerable apprehension and impatience at nine months pregnant:

[Real-time account] 'Impending labour exercises my mind somewhat, fairly cataclysmic ... You wonder physically what it's going to be like, actually giving birth ... And I suppose a little bit of fear about whether you will come through it intact ... You also feel impatient with your sort of lumbering body.'

Her retrospective account of the same time period, written five months after the birth of the child, presents a more singularly positive picture:

'There is a sense of anticipation – not animated excitement, just gentle waiting ... There is a dreamlike quality about this last stage of the proceedings with the waiting, and the heavy, lumbering movement which has a grace of its own, despite the discomfort. I am a lady in waiting.'

Here, a contemporaneous account of uncertainty and some anxiety is retrospectively reconstructed as one of idyllic calm. Clare even uses the same term – 'lumbering' – to describe her body, but it is reinterpreted more positively.

This is typical of the discrepancies found in the women's case studies which suggest considerable reflexive reconstruction taking place. The women, when looking back to the pregnancy after the child is born, construct a story of what it was like, a story differing in several respects from the one they told as the pregnancy was actually unfolding. One can then, of course, speculate about the reasons for such reconstruction. It may represent a coping strategy for dealing with unpleasant events, a wish to think well of the period which produced the child she now has, and so forth (see Smith, 1994a, for further discussion).

I would argue that this study helps to bring reflexive theory and practice together. The reflexive self as envisaged by Mead, Gergen and Giddens is realised within a particular research design. When seen at nine months pregnant, the woman presented an account of self in relation to the pregnancy. Later, thinking back to, and reporting on, the same chronological time point, she presents a different conception of self. Thus, the model of 'self at nine months pregnant' held by the woman at one time point is, at a subsequent time point, radically reconstructed and this illustrates, and depends on the existence of, the reflexive self as posited earlier. It is only the woman's ability to reflect back on herself that allows her to revise the conception of that self that she has. Without this ability, the biographical record would remain essentially stable.

Methodologically, while examining only retrospective accounts of pregnancy would have allowed one to speculate on possible constructive strategies employed by the woman, the extent of the examination would have been severely prescribed. By comparing contemporaneous and retrospective accounts and examining discrepancies between them, the reconstructive strategies are highlighted. We are able to witness self-reconstruction in action, or, to use Gidden's phrase quoted earlier, 'self-identity ... as interpreted reflexively by the agent'. The approach outlined in this section also clearly links to the growing field of narrative psychology (see Crossley, 2000; Murray, 2003).

Reflexive analysis and dialogical interpretation

In the practice of doing a research project it is possible to push further some implications of the reflexive thesis. If one's view of a person is as a self-reconstructing reflexive agent and given that one's respondent will therefore be doing this reflexing anyway, why not explicitly enlist her or him as a co-researcher in the project? This way one can be seen to be addressing and engaging with reflexivity at a number of intra- and interpersonal levels. This model has usually been associated with the humanistically inspired co-operative inquiry approach (see Reason, 2003). However, it is a move which can follow logically from the reflexive thesis whether one tends more to an essentialist or a constructionist theory of persons. Mulkay (1985) describes a form of dialogical analysis whereby he engaged in an ongoing exchange – corresponding with a scientist whose work had been the topic of a sociological research project by Mulkay himself. He writes of this approach:

> 'For example why not create an analysis in the form of a dialogue with one, or more, of the actual participants? This kind of analysis, as far as I know, has not been tried before. It would be a stringent test of one's analysis to offer it for close scrutiny and comment to those responsible for the original texts ... In the course of such an analysis, one could not be continually concerned with one's own textuality. There would be no alternative to projecting one's claims upon participants' own textual products. However, one's analysis would then become a text available to participants for deconstruction and textual analysis. In this way, by abandoning the analyst's usual assumption of interpretative privilege, one could enlist participants' help in revealing one's own textuality, whilst at the same time digging more deeply into their interpretative capacities and your own' (1985, p.76).

Mulkay's suggestion seems to envisage a model of doing research which derives from and corresponds to a theory of persons as reflexive, social and mentating beings. Finding ways to study such beings is indeed likely to require creating more sophisticated and dynamic methodologies, but as Allport (1963) notes, 'we should adapt our methods so far as we can to the object and not define the object in terms of our faulty methods' (1963, p.28).

Mulkay recognises that research involves simultaneous engagement with persons and with texts. He also recognises the reflexive work researcher and respondent bring to this encounter, their equal engagement in the activity reflected in the notion of enlisting the respondent as co-analyst. Obviously this attempt at a more negotiated form of analysis will only be possible and appropriate in certain research projects. Researchers attempting such dialogic exercises also need to reflect carefully on how the issues of power, responsibility and ownership are being played out.

Within the motherhood project, I engaged in a form of co-operative, reflexive analysis. Once I had collected all the first-order data from a woman and done some preliminary analysis, I visited her again and discussed the material with her. This conversation was itself tape-recorded and used in subsequent second-order analysis which was incorporated into the final write-up. An abbreviated version of one example of this form of dialogical analysis is provided below; the full version can be seen in Smith (1994b).

Angela, another participant in the motherhood project, kept a diary throughout the pregnancy in which she recorded any thoughts that came to her about the pregnancy and how it was affecting her. At four months pregnant, Angela started writing about a pregnant neighbour who was three months further ahead in her pregnancy. At six months, Angela writes:

'The baby is lovely. I saw her on Monday and Sara came home from hospital on Thursday ... I really feel maternal when I hold the baby.'

When reading the first sentence, it struck me as ambiguous. Which baby? Angela's or the neighbour's? This fleeting uncertainty is removed as soon as one reaches the second sentence which marks the reference as to the neighbour's child. Why did I feel the first sentence was ambiguous? This echoes a whole series of previous references by Angela to her own baby as *the baby*, cueing anaphoric resonance here. Reading the same abbreviated form in 'the baby is lovely', I perhaps thought Angela was referring to seeing her baby on a scan.

Angela appears to feel considerable involvement in her neighbour's pregnancy and this seems to facilitate increasing engagement with her own pregnancy (as she makes explicit at the end of the above extract). I may have thought, therefore, that the ambiguities reflected this connection: the appearance of another baby has helped awaken excitement about her own; the close timing means attention is divided between the two pregnancies and this split attention may be leaking out in the ambiguous referent, *the baby*. This became a topic for the dialogic analysis session with Angela at the end of the project. I first showed her the above diary entry without any comment or interpretation from me. She responded:

'Every time I thought "I don't know what I'm going to do", I could go over there and, you know, that could be my baby for ten minutes.'

Then after I gave a brief presentation of my interpretation, as outlined above, Angela responded:

'Now you've read it out, anyone would assume I was talking about my own ... I felt at that time that any baby was mine ... I didn't think of it as being anyone else's when I picked it up.'

Angela's comments suggest the ambiguous identity referents are even more significant than I had originally considered. So powerful is the bond with the other baby that she (and indeed any baby) can, in a sense, become her own. Thus the ambiguity of 'the baby is lovely' becomes entirely appropriate because it can be referring to any baby but by the same token any baby it does refer to is Angela's.

There are two levels of reflexive analysis occurring here. During the first part of the final discussion with Angela, I merely presented some of her account back to her. This then became the stimulus for second-order commentary by her as she reflected now on what she had written in the diary. Thus, the material is acting to encourage a natural propensity for reflexivity on the part of the participant.

Then in the second part, the reflexive analysis expands to include the interpersonal level. I gave my reading to Angela and she used this to reflect further on her perception and she provides a further elaboration on the original interpretation. This in turn influenced my own interpretative activity. I would suggest that we were, during this exchange, engaging in a dialogical form of reflexive analysis and, to use Mulkay's terms, 'digging more deeply into' our 'interpretative capacities'.

This, then, has provided another illustration of reflexivity theory reflected in practice. An approach to research has been influenced by a reflexive model of persons. The analytic dialogue which ensues is both capitalising on, and illustrating the facility for, reflexivity on the part of both participant and investigator and the interaction itself is a form of interpersonal reflexivity. It is worth pointing out that the dialogical reflexivity illustrated here is different from 'member/respondent validation' which has traditionally been held up as a hallmark of quality control in qualitative research. The aim with the process outlined here is to include the participant in the analytic process, not to ask the participant to state whether they agree or disagree with the researcher's reading. For useful discussions on current views on validity in qualitative research see Yardley (2000) and Elliott *et al.* (1999).

Summary

In conclusion, this chapter has attempted to illustrate how a more central role for reflexivity can be afforded within psychological theory and practice. Taking reflexivity as a central concern for a psychology of persons, I have explored the linkage between theoretical models and methodological designs and offered proposals for how reflexivity can inform psychological practice. Reflexivity has been conceived as operating at both intra- and interpersonal levels, and examples of studies of each of these have been included in order to illustrate more closely how the reflexive thesis might play out in specific psychological research strategies. Of course, these are not the only ways in which reflexivity becomes manifest and can be harnessed in research projects; rather the aim has been to detail two particular practices

References

Allport, G. (1947) *The Use of Personal Documents in Psychological Science*. Social Science Research Council, New York.

Allport, G. (1963) *Pattern and Growth in Personality*. Holt Rinehart & Winston, London.

Burkitt, I. (1991) *Social Selves*. Sage Publications, London.

Butler, J. (1990) *Gender Trouble: Feminism and the Subversion of Identity*. Routledge, New York.

Crossley, M. (2000) *Introducing Narrative Psychology*. Open University Press, Milton Keynes.

Datan, N., Rodeheaver, D. & Hughes, F. (1987) Adult development and aging. *Annual Review of Psychology*, **38**, 153–80.

Denscombe, M. (2001) Uncertain identities and health-risking behaviour. *British Journal of Sociology*, **52**, 157–77.

Elliott, R., Fischer, C. & Rennie, D. (1999) Evolving guidelines for publication of qualitative research studies in psychology and related fields. *British Journal of Clinical Psychology*, **38**, 215–29.

Gergen, K. (1980) The emerging crisis in life-span developmental psychology. In *Life-span Development and Behaviour*, Volume 3 (Baltes, P. & Brim, O., eds). Academic Press, New York.

Giddens, A. (1991) *Modernity and Self-Identity*. Polity Press, Cambridge.

Gleitman, B. (1999) *Psychology*, 5th edn. Norton, New York.

Manning, C. & Loftus, E. (1996) Eyewitness testimony and memory distortion. *Japanese Psychological Research*, **38**, 5–13.

Mead, G.H. (1934) *Mind, Self and Society*. Chicago University Press, Chicago.

Mulkay, M. (1985) *The Word and the World*. Allen and Unwin, London.

Murray, M. (2003) Narrative psychology. In *Qualitative Psychology* (Smith, J.A., ed.). Sage Publications, London.

Pavis, S., Cuningham-Burley, S. & Amos, A. (1998) Health related behavioural change in context. *Social Science and Medicine*, **47**, 1407–18.

Plummer, K. (2001) *Documents of Life 2: An Invitation to Critical Humanism*. Sage Publications, London.

Reason, P. (2003, in press) Co-operative inquiry. In *Qualitative Psychology* (Smith, J.A., ed.). Sage Publications, London.

Smith, J.A. (1994a) Reconstructing selves: an analysis of discrepancies between women's contemporaneous and retrospective accounts of the transition to motherhood. *British Journal of Psychology*, **85**, 371–92.

Smith, J.A. (1994b) Towards reflexive practice: engaging participants as co-researchers or co-analysts in psychological inquiry. *Journal of Community & Applied Social Psychology*, **4**, 253–60.

Smith, J.A. (2003) Interpretative phenomenological analysis. In *Qualitative Psychology* (Smith, J.A. ed.). Sage Publications, London.

Wyatt, F. (1964) The reconstruction of the individual and of the collective past. In *The Study of Lives: Essays on Personality in Honor of Henry A Murray* (White, R.W., ed.). Atherton Press, New York.

Yardley, L. (2000) Dilemmas in qualitative health research. *Psychology and Health*, **15**, 215–28.

CHAPTER 14

Researcher as storyteller and performer: parallels with playback theatre

Nick Rowe

Positioning the self: author's story

My passion for playback theatre began in 1995 when I joined the York Playback Theatre Company. Playback theatre is a form of improvised theatre in which members of the audience tell personal stories to a company of experienced actors and musicians and watch as it is spontaneously 'played back' to them. The York company is made up of therapists, educators and professional actors. We have performed to public audiences, students, conferences, 'users' of mental health services, patients in hospices and guests at a wedding.

My doctoral research into 'playback' began in 1997. It seemed to me then, and it still does now, that researching playback gave me the opportunity to combine the 'professional' and the 'personal' in ways that would enrich both aspects of my life. In my professional life, as a dramatherapist and lecturer in occupational therapy, I have been interested in the therapist as someone who enables the client to tell and shape their story. In playback theatre I have been able to tell my own personal stories and see them shaped by the actors into theatre. I have tried to combine these insights and experiences in my research so that the personal sheds light on the professional and vice versa.

A major challenge in my research has been to write about playback theatre in a way that is sympathetic to the form. I aim to resist the contention that what happens in an improvised performance is inexpressible and beyond the grasp of words – a view which, it seems to me, often only leads to a kind of sloppy mysticism. In an improvised theatre practice such as playback there are always multiple viewpoints – so I try to write from the *inside* and the *outside* of playback theatre and all the places in between. I strive, reflexively, to make each perspective susceptible to other viewpoints so that the polyphony of the playback form is maintained.

Introduction

In this chapter, I introduce you to the guiding metaphor of my research method – the research process as playback theatre process. I will try to illustrate how it is possible to see the research task as being analogous with that of playback storyteller and performer. I will explain how this guiding metaphor has allowed me to stay as close as I can to the *lived experience* of playback theatre. To these ends I present some passages describing moments in playback theatre and also a series of boxes containing reflections on my research.

Researching playback theatre: opportunities and challenges

'The actors sit facing the audience.
The teller sits on stage next to the "conductor" whose task is to help them tell their story.
Their story must be an autobiographical one.
If the teller casts an actor he or she stands.
When the story is told the conductor briefly summarises the story and says "Let's watch". This is the cue for the actors to begin.
They improvise the story without consultation with each other.
When the "enactment" finishes the teller is briefly asked to comment on what they have seen.
This is playback theatre.'

Playback theatre is an encounter between the 'performer', the 'teller', their 'story' and the 'audience'. In this encounter the performer spontaneously responds to the teller's personal story within the dramatic forms of playback theatre. The performer's response to the teller's story draws upon the former's personal experience, their grasp of human narrative, their psychobiological response and their understanding of dramatic form.

In the course of my research into playback theatre I have been struck by the fertile reciprocity that is available when one holds the roles of researcher and playback actor in simultaneous awareness. Like playback theatre, the research task may also be conceived of as an encounter. It is an encounter between the researcher, the participant and their story and the audience who will eventually consume the work. The researcher's response may also draw upon personal experience, narrative understanding, cognitive and even somatic response, and an understanding of methodological forms and approaches.

It has seemed to me that in exploring the interconnectedness of research topic and methodological approach, I am more likely to achieve a methodology that is sympathetic and responsive to my area of research. Another way of putting this is to say that field and method need to be held in a *reflexive relationship* with each other. My task, as a researcher studying playback theatre, has therefore been to devise a methodological approach that is congruent with the playback process itself, one that possesses some of the qualities of playback theatre – spontaneity, flexibility and an acute awareness of a range of voices or modes of expression. This chapter explores this rich relationship between research method and play-back theatre – expecting that one will shed light on the other. In order to do this I will ask you, the reader, to consider two metaphors of the research task – the researcher as *storyteller* and the researcher as *actor* – both of which, in the spirit of my argument, derive from playback theatre practice. Before doing this, how-ever, I want to mention two complex issues which I have had to negotiate during my research on playback theatre – two issues which I believe confront all qua-litative researchers: ephemerality and researcher as involved participant.

The research of improvised theatre practice involves significant methodological problems and opportunities. Theatre is a live event, taking place in the here and now. Attempts to preserve its 'liveness' run into significant difficulties. Memory of the performance decays quickly and forms of video and audio recording cannot retain the vivacity of the moment. The particular contexts of the event – the perceptual sets of the participants and the particular patterns of meaning that emerge during the performance – cannot be preserved in their totality. Specifi-cally, playback theatre derives its energy from relationships in the here and now – relationships between performers, spectators and teller. Our memory of these relationships is always partial (Clifford, 1986) in both senses of the word – it records only 'part of' any experience and it is always, and unavoidably, sub-jective. In order to respond to the challenge of ephemerality, a method that is emergent, improvisational and deeply responsive to the moment is required, in other words, a method consonant with playback theatre practice itself.

In addition, the naïve view that the researcher is separated from the field of research by objectivity and protective protocols is, to say the least, problematic for research into playback theatre. There are significant methodological problems for the researcher who is immersed in the field of research and has relationships with professional and personal 'research subjects' that extend far beyond the research focus. There is, to use the language of anthropology, the danger of 'going native' and of 'becoming the phenomenon'. This is illustrated by some reflections (see Box 11.1) written at the outset of my study.

It is a question of how the researcher is positioned in what might be called the processual flux of the research. At the very least, the question suggests two roles: the *critical observer*, positioned outside the field, and the *engaged participant*, positioned inside. From each position the research field will be perceived and constructed differently, and, of central importance, the voice or register of the research presented from these different positions will vary. The register delivered by the insider immersed in the life of the ensemble and the empathies and inti-macies of playback acting will be of a different quality from that delivered from

> ### Box 14.1   Problems and opportunities of shared history
>
> This group with whom I intend to conduct research have a shared history with me spanning two years before the commencement of this research. They have played my stories and I have played theirs. They know some of my history and vice versa. This seems a most important set of relationships to acknowledge and position my research with regard to. Many of the traditional roles of the researcher are therefore unavailable to me. I am a committed and very involved member of the company. The company plays an important part in how I describe myself and construct my identity. Rather like Jules-Rossette (1978), who converted to the religious group she was studying, I am an active and 'believing' member of this group I aim to study. This raises a whole series of methodological problems and opportunities that I will need to address.

the outside. These different registers need to be identified and distinguished. In my experience of conducting this research, there is a complex range of positions along the continuum of 'insider' to 'outsider' and these will need to be heard. The task is to maintain both positions – inside and outside the research field – and to render the voices that may be heard from these positions.

The challenge of ephemerality and the problems and opportunities of being an involved participant call for a method that is as sympathetic to playback theatre as possible. As I have suggested above, in order to achieve this I have sought to hold method and field in *simultaneous relationship* by using the practice of playback theatre as a metaphorical device to structure the method. In the section that follows I will consider two key aspects of playback practice: the telling of autobiographical stories and the demands of playback acting. This gives me two rich metaphors to explore – the researcher as storyteller and the researcher as performer.

The researcher as storyteller

'All we sociologists have are stories. Some from other people, some from us, some from our interaction with others. What matters is to understand how and where the stories are produced, which stories they are and how we can put them to honest and intelligent use in theorising about social life' (Silverman, 1997, p.111).

Research involves the telling of a story. Paul Atkinson (1990) writes of the 'ethnographer's tale' as often being presented as the story of a quest or a journey of discovery. What are the characteristics of this particular research story? It is a story told to a particular audience, one that involves some degree of self-disclosure and one that requires to be told in a range of voices. My research story is emergent, improvised; always partial and inflected by my motivations. What follows is a discussion of key features pertaining to storytelling – in both playback theatre and qualitative research generally.

Here is a brief reflection on preparing to tell a story in the context of playback theatre:

> 'Imagine the teller, "heavy" with his or her story, taking the dangerous path from the auditorium to the stage. To tell a story in public is a risky thing to do – she perhaps fears that she will not be able to tell the story well enough. She is also aware of the audience: "Will they accept my story? Will they think me foolish for telling it? Will I reveal more than I intend?"'

The telling of a research story is something like this. The researcher often experiences the same kind of 'performance anxiety', the same sense of risk. My early journal notes suggest two contrasting experiences at the beginning of the research – a kind of 'puppy dog' enthusiasm in which I was unaware of the deep waters I was getting into and a persistent anxiety that I was not up to the job. Telling a personal story in a playback performance and writing qualitative research both involve a kind of exposure to the judgement of others. Even now I am conscious of the responses my research story might elicit – from the academic community for whom it is being written, from the playback company about whom I am writing (and with whom I have a committed set of relationships which will continue after the story is told), and from the wider playback theatre who will be interested in my work as one of the first on the subject. Like the teller who comes forward to tell a story at a performance I am aware of these audiences and their possible conflicting expectations.

As an example of how the writer's awareness of conflicting audiences may shed light on the research field, I offer in Box 14.2 a description of my feelings of discomfort that accompanied the task of critically examining some of the writing of Jonathan Fox and Jo Salas, the most prolific writers in the playback field.

Box 14.2　Feeling uncomfortable

A sense of betrayal has accompanied the writing of this section. I have almost exclusively quoted from Jonathan Fox and Jo Salas and, although this is not surprising since they have written significantly more than any other in the field, it does produce in me a rather uneasy feeling. The selections from their work have been chosen to bring the writing into question and to expose playback's discourse to a critique. I have met and worked with both of them and respect their work. This process is made more uncomfortable because of that.

It is important for me to acknowledge these feelings since they shed light on the particular intimacy of the playback community and perhaps even its cloistered nature. My feelings also highlight the central position held by these two figures. In other words a heightened awareness of the storyteller/writer's audience reveals possible dynamics for exploration in the research field.

In actually recounting the (research) story, the narrator should ideally recognise multiple speaking positions.

'The teller begins to tell her story to the conductor. As she does so she becomes aware of the many layers that may require expression and the different styles that may be used in the telling. Should she tell the story with the emotional weight of someone inside the experience? Or should she dispassionately report the story, as if standing outside it?'

In qualitative research the researcher too is aware of the multiple subject positions or registers that need to be heard. As James Clifford (1986, p.103) emphasises: 'The staging and valuing of multiple and allegorical registers or "voices" becomes an important area ... interrupting the privileged monotone of scientific representation'. As the teller of this story, I recognise the importance of reflecting as many voices as possible in the research. It requires a fragmentary approach that favours narrative over theory and a fluid, dynamic writing style over one-dimensional meta-narratives. It obliges me as James Clifford writes: 'to find diverse ways of rendering negotiated realities as multi-subjective, power-laden and incongruent' (1986, p.15).

In the following extract (Box 14.3) I bring to bear a number of registers and voices to the task of examining a performance sequence. The teller had recounted the onset of a depression, which caused him to hide away from others and to become obsessed with persecutory thoughts. In the left-hand column I try to describe what happened as 'coolly' as possible. In the right-hand column, I note, as the actor cast to play the teller, some personal process of which I was aware at the time. I follow this with a brief analysis, drawing upon another actor's experience.

In the moments before an enactment begins the actor searches for some idea, image, feeling or physical impulse that will help him or her in the performance. In this instance, it was my own memories of a relatively mild depressive phase in my late twenties and the physical feelings that accompanied that which presented themselves to me as I stood listening to the story. Box 14.4 offers another example where my reactions intertwined with others.

In this section I have tried to bring together a range of subject positions or registers – a relatively detached description of events and an 'insider's' account of the dramatic sequence. I have also employed the words of another actor on the process of decision making in playback performance and my personal voice in response to her words. The aim of both these examples was to give insights into the process of playback acting in such a way that the polyphony of the form is maintained.

Box 14.3   Objective and personal descriptions

Description

The teller went on to say that during his period of 'depression' his mother had died. It was a time in which he was overwhelmed and distressed by persecutory thoughts. He spent days in his room, afraid to come out. He described how, after his mother's death, he moved back to the city where he had lived before and gradually began to improve with the help of family and friends. When asked to give a title to his story he offered 'Deliverance'. On invitation he gave an image of himself on top of a mountain with friends looking down and celebrating his deliverance.

Personal Process

As the actor cast to play the teller, I feel a strong identification with him – I recognise the obsession with persecutory thoughts, the wish to hide and I think I know what he means by the word 'deliverance'. I am reminded of a period in my life when I had similar experiences.

The film *Deliverance* comes to mind, but in this moment I can't remember what it was about – something to do with boats and white water rapids.

Box 14.4   Encountering one's own story

An actor describes her choice of black and white cloth during a performance. The teller had described a time in her life which was particularly drab and unhappy. Afterwards the actor told me: 'In my mind was a line that I thought I might use at some point and that was, "a lot of surviving but not much thriving". I remember a few years ago reading a book, which said something like "Yes you have survived but have you thrived?" Because she chose me, this phrase was going through my mind and black and white seemed, to me, to be more about surviving than thriving. I didn't think of this at the time but I went through a time a few years ago when the world seemed black and white and had no colour.'

After my discussion with her I write: 'Why did I feel tearful when she told me this? It was the integrity of her description and my own recognition of the way playback acting can be. It can be an encounter with one's own story through the teller's.'

Another consideration for the storyteller, in both playback theatre and qualitative research, concerns how much of oneself should be revealed in the performance and writing. In the presence of an audience we must decide how much to tell. We might be anxious that we will reveal too much and we ask, 'Will the audience be sympathetic to my story? Am I going to embarrass myself? Will they think me foolish? Will I embarrass them?'

As a writer committed to a reflexive approach, I have faced these dilemmas and have needed to make difficult decisions about how much to reveal of myself in the writing. During the time that I have been working on this research both of my parents have died. As a member of the company I have told my story of their death and watched it 'played back'. As a researcher I have reported on this and allowed it to shed light on the playback process. In the following extract (Box 14.5) I describe an enactment of the story of the day my father died. In my research the extract is used to illustrate how memory is created and changed through a playback enactment. When I told this story in rehearsal, I described to the actor's how, immediately after my father died, I caught sight of my daughter cycling in the bright sunshine wearing a red coat.

Box 14.5 A personal story

I told the story of my father's dying day at a playback rehearsal in early October 1998 – only weeks after the event itself. I told the actors about the red coat and cast one of them to be my daughter. This actor, swathed in red cloth, circled the stage throughout the enactment, making a very strong impression on me, to such an extent that this is now the only part of the enactment that I remember. It is clear that the performance altered my memory of the day my Dad died, or at the very least, pushed to the foreground the red coat aspect of it. Subsequent retellings have always stressed that aspect, arguably far more forcefully that would have been the case if I had not viewed that performance. As it happens I would contend that this has enriched my narrative, giving me an image that previously did not have the resonance it now has. It is clearly the case that the performance has contributed to the fictionalising of one aspect of the story – literally reinforcing what I later discovered to be fictional – that the coat was pink and not red.

The researcher as playback actor

As well as storyteller, the researcher may also be analogously seen as an actor in a playback performance.

> 'The actor listens carefully to the story as it is told, knowing that soon she will have to find a spontaneous response to it. She tries to relate the story to her own experience or to those whom she knows. She tries to be aware of her body's responses to the story and to the emotions that it invokes in her. She knows that, to some extent, she will "interpret" the story, put a "spin" on it and that can be a daunting responsibility. But perhaps most importantly she really doesn't know what will happen – the enactment will emerge – that's the risk and the excitement.
>
> The playback actor is poised at the moment of the telling of the story with

senses attuned to the teller and the story. The actor feels she knows this story but struggles against a temptation simply to tell her own version. The actor must find a balance between the surprise of the new – an idiosyncratic story told for the first time – and the recognition of the "familiarity" of the story and the personal and cultural resonances within it.'

This *creative balance* between familiarity and strangeness seems an important one for research. It is, after all, impossible to perceive an object as totally new '…one does not start (or ought not) intellectually empty-handed' (Geertz, 1993, p.27). This is, of course, particularly true for the writer as an already experienced member of a playback company. However it is important, as far as I can, to see the world as 'anthropologically strange' (Hammersley & Atkinson, 1983, p.12) – to see the 'normal' as unfamiliar. It seems to me, that the only way to maintain some sense of the strangeness of the field is, paradoxically, to maintain a high degree of reflexivity in acknowledging its familiarity.

One way to render the familiar strange is to pay special awareness to those moments when the 'unusual' happens, since the unusual alerts us to what is usual. In Box 14.6 an unusual moment in a performance leads to an important insight into the playback process that has subsequently been influential in the development of my thesis.

Box 14.6   An insight

A woman told a story that concerned her first panic attack. When the story was enacted, one of the actors stood behind the actor cast as the teller. She gave some verbal expression to her (the teller's) inner feelings and thoughts. When the enactment was over, a member of the audience asked the conductor, 'What did that woman mean when she stood behind the person playing the teller?'

This is a rare moment in playback theatre. It is unusual for members of the audience to ask for explanations of what is happening onstage. The fact that this event was uncommon in the experience of the company was clear by the hesitation of the conductor in addressing the question. Eventually, the conductor replied, 'What do you think she was doing?' The questioner answered that she was speaking some of the thoughts of the teller's actor. Later, the conductor told me, 'I didn't want to get into a discussion about meaning and technique.' This moment is an interesting one since it reveals one of the unspoken conventions of playback theatre – that discussions over meaning, interpretation or the dramatic choices of actors are kept to a minimum.

An actor must also be able to embody the moment.

'During the enactment the actor has often little idea of what to do. In fact it is often better to not know what will happen next. She must rely on her *awareness* of her body, her emotions, the here and now relationships in space and the actions of the other actors. She does not just listen to the manifest words but also responds to the physicality of the teller, the tone of delivery and the impact this has on her physical, affective and cognitive awareness. She tries to be aware of the internal stimuli that will impel her to action.'

To what extent can we speak of the researcher apprehending the research field in this way? There are two points I wish to make here. Firstly, the importance of the personal awareness of the researcher. Stanley and Wise forcefully stress this in their argument for radical feminist research when they argue that, 'all research must be concerned with the experiences and consciousness of the researcher as an integral part of the research process' (1993, p.58).

Secondly, the playback actor will be aware not just of the spoken word but also of other sensory input received from the teller. Is it possible to conceive of research that engages all the senses? A researcher writing ethnography must, it seems to me, record what is seen, heard, touched, smelt and tasted (Okely, 1994). The following sequence in Box 14.7 (taken from the same enactment described in Box 14.3) illustrates the use of somatic experience in playback acting. The sequence illustrates the process of 'somatic identification' in playback acting and was used as data to discuss that subject. The process, by which the actor identifies with the teller through physical sensations, is one that is often crucial in improvised playback performance. The sequence demonstrates how the participant researcher apprehends the field through somatic engagement with it. The somatic experiences I describe give an impetus to the actor and an insight into the dynamics of playback acting for the researcher.

Box 14.7 Somatic experiencing

When the conductor said 'Let's watch', I waited by the side of the stage while the musician played and other actors took cloth.

As I stood, I noticed my breathing becoming more heavy and that there were 'churning' feelings in my stomach.

Although I did not know how the enactment would develop, I knew that these physical experiences would provide me with movement and sound to begin the piece. One way of putting this is that what I would do would come from the breathing and the stomach.

I worked on 'holding on to' these feelings.

An actor inevitably interprets the story.

> 'The actor knows that she cannot avoid interpreting the teller's story. Every movement, every inflection of the facial muscles, every word that is spoken makes meaning. Nor can she avoid meaning being attributed to the enactment by the teller and the audience. There is no neutral place on stage.'

It is much the same in qualitative research. Through the structuring of their material, through the choice of thematic organisation, the writer is involved in acts of interpretation and, in common with the playback actor, the researcher cannot totally control the meanings that will be attributed to the work. There is no neutral space in qualitative research writing. Researchers must, therefore, take responsibility for their interpretative role, as must the playback actor. The researcher accepts, like the playback actor, that his or her response will inevitably be influenced by preference and personal and cultural horizons.

The researcher, like the playback actor, needs to be aware of this interpretative system and how this is derived from a store of *cultural stories*. These cultural stories and discourse modes are, of course, embedded in patterns of mutually dependent communal life. Just as the actor depends on the community of the ensemble with whom he plays and the communal life which gives meaning to what he does, so the researcher is dependent on the research culture and the wider culture for the generation of meaning.

Finally, an actor must attempt to 'let go'.

> 'As the actor begins it is likely that she will not know how the enactment will develop. Despite her anxiety, she knows from her experience that the story will emerge if she "trusts the process". It can be a struggle to believe in that, however. She is tempted to "force" things.'

Keith Johnstone puts this in a different way, but essentially expresses what I want to say: 'We have an idea that art is self-expression – which historically is weird. An artist used to be seen as a medium through which something else operated' (1985, p.78). Is it possible to see the research writer as a 'medium' through which the research story will unfold? While recognising the danger of recourse to the mystical, I nevertheless think that these notions may be helpful in conceiving the research task. Of course we are speaking here about improvisation and spontaneity in the research process.

In the extract that follows (see Box 14.8) I attempt to write 'freely' about the interpretative role of playback actor and the dangers of being lost in 'metaphorical jungles' and the sheer playfulness of the genre. The extract also illustrates how research insight may emerge through the writing and how there may be a rich interplay between reflexive views on the research field and on the act of research itself.

Box 14.8 Becoming lost

For an actor there is a danger of becoming lost in the endless folds and turns (the etymological root of trope) of tropes – a trope-ical jungle!

As a playback actor I enter this trope-ical jungle; I become fascinated by its strange exotic fruits, the myriad colours and gradations of light that play upon the leaves. Beginning to forget why I am there (leaving the story far behind like the swimmer, the shore), I meet other actors. Together we play, enjoying the twists and turns that this jungle offers. We might say that, under the spotlight, under the gaze of the audience we regress until – like children stopped in their play – we find a way to end, blinking from the harsh light of reality.

This happens in playback performances sometimes, usually when the actors have not listened to the story or it is unclear or the story is deeply introspective and has no 'grounding' in real life events.

The writer too can be lost – building castles of theoretical speculation or placing fondly held beliefs under the glare of inspection until they begin to slip and slide and the writer loses his footing.

Like the playback actor, the researcher must trust the research process. He or she must resist the temptation to force meaning but instead allow it to emerge from a deep immersion in the material and the experience of the research field. Another way of putting this is to say that the researcher requires a willingness to relinquish some control over the process. As Kleinmann and Copp write, 'Qualitative researchers only gain control of their projects by first allowing themselves to lose it' (1993, p.3).

Summary

The aim of this chapter has been to explore a range of methodological issues and experiences that arise in both playback theatre and qualitative research. Both present challenges in terms of processing what is happening and for writing up. What is required is an approach that acknowledges the ephemeral and immediate, while also remaining sensitive to the research field itself. My examination of researching playback has developed out of the reflexive interplay of field and method. My strategy has been to use playback theatre as a metaphor for the research process and I have considered two key metaphors to that end: the researcher as storyteller and the researcher as actor. Holding the research task and playback theatre in simultaneous awareness has provided me with an active precept to judge the quality of my work and to guide me through the inevitable 'cloud of unknowing' that characterises the writing task.

References

Atkinson, P. (1990) *The Ethnographer's Imagination: Textual Constructions of Reality.* Routledge, London.

Clifford, J. (1986) Introduction: partial truths. In *Writing Culture: The Poetics and Politics of Ethnography* (Clifford, J. & Marcus, G., eds). University of California Press, CA.

Geertz, C. (1993) *The Interpretation of Cultures.* Fontana, London.

Hammersley, M. & Atkinson, P. (1983) *Ethnography: Principles and Practice.* Routledge, London.

Johnstone, K. (1985) *Impro: Improvisation and the Theatre.* Methuen, London.

Jules-Rossette, B. (1978) Cited in Hammersley, M. & Atkinson, P. (1983) *Ethnography: Principles and Practice.* Routledge, London.

Kleinmann, S. & Copp, M. (1993) *Emotions and Fieldwork.* Sage Publications, London.

Okely, J. (1994) Thinking through fieldwork. In *Analysing Qualitative Data* (Bryman, A. & Burgess, R., eds). Routledge, London.

Silverman, D. (1997) *Qualitative Research: Theory, Method and Practice.* Sage Publications, London.

Stanley, L. & Wise, S. (1993) *Breaking Out Again.* Routledge, London.

CHAPTER 15

Using reflexivity to loosen theoretical and organisational knots within participatory action research

Majella McFadden and Alison McCamley

Positioning the selves: authors' stories

We both lecture and research in psychology at Sheffield Hallam University and have worked together on projects where qualitative methods and reflexive practices figure prominently.

The appeal of qualitative approaches for us lies in their potential to tap the complexity and messiness of human experiences. They provide opportunities to interrogate the assumptions and values threaded through research, including the political spaces that the researcher occupies at different times. Throughout our research experiences reflexivity has enabled us to weave our way through differing layers of theoretical awareness, communication styles and subject positions. Of course, the utility of reflexivity as a research tool for those working within the broadly defined contexts of qualitative research is well-documented in ongoing debates (Wilkinson, 1988; Denzin & Lincoln, 1994; Gough, 1999).

In this chapter we focus on the multiple ways in which reflexive practices facilitated the management and development of a participatory action research project we recently worked on. The Sheffield Young People's Sexual Health Peer Research Project consisted of a complex matrix of research participants including young people, statutory and voluntary agencies, peer researchers, research and development workers and social research practitioners within Sheffield. Throughout the two years of our involvement with this project, we became increasingly aware of the many ways that using reflexive practices enabled us to engage with and loosen – rather than unravel – a number of tight theoretical and organisational knots. In particular, we argue that reflexivity:

- Allows an exploration of, and a means of challenging, the ways in which assumptions, professional identities and political positions influence research.
- Generates a 'public' dialogue on subjectivity within the research matrix through which others' understandings and practices relating to research can be explored (in this instance, the significant others were the research and development workers and the young people with whom we are co-researching).

Contd.

Positioning the selves: authors' stories *Contd.*

- Enables the refining of research practices by functioning as a means of communication through which the research project could be organised, developed and evaluated.
- Enhances the development of critical social theory.

There a number of ways of tracking the influence of the researcher(s) and the research process on the findings produced. Banister *et al.* (1994) suggest keeping a diary that details the ways in which the thoughts and experiences of researchers shift throughout the research process. Whilst recognising the complexities associated with the fluid and fragmented nature of subjectivity (Wetherell & Maybin, 1996; Seale, 1999), this chapter draws on the diaries of the university-based researchers and the research and development workers, as well as documented discussions in various group meetings (research team, steering/advisory groups) pertaining to the research process and the production of interim and final reports.

The Sheffield Young People's Sexual Health Peer Research Project: theoretical and organisational context

The Sheffield Young People's Sexual Health Project (August 1999–August 2001) was funded by the UK National Lottery (Community Fund) and structured through a consortium of young people from Sheffield, host agencies, voluntary and statutory agencies and Sheffield Hallam University (see Figure 15.1). Essentially, the project set out to explore the meanings and contexts within which young people defined and practised sexual health so that future resources and services could be more relevant to their needs. The research team consisted of thirty young people, two research and development workers, three adult volunteers and two university-based researchers.

The project was situated within the now familiar critique of positivism and the increasing realisation among qualitative researchers that the research they undertake is not a value-free inquiry but, rather, a socially constructed account co-produced between the researcher and others participating in the research process (Reason, 1988; Wilkinson, 1988; Denzin & Lincoln, 1994). Within this context, then, reflexive practices are placed centre stage, as there is an increasing onus on the social researcher to make explicit the ways in which personal, interpersonal and organisational dynamics influence the direction and outcome of research.

Furthermore, the project discussed in this chapter is situated within wider social and political contexts that increasingly prioritise (and reward, with respect to funding) the need for researchers to capture the voices of so-called vulnerable

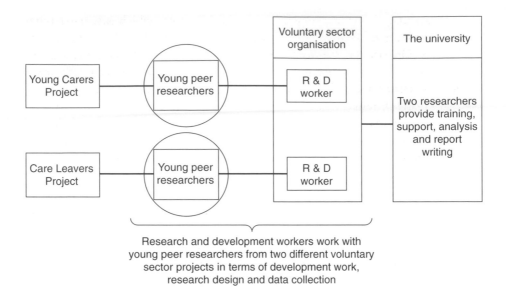

Fig. 15.1 Groups and agencies involved.

or marginalised groups in society. In particular, this is reflected within a health promotion context in Britain where there is an emphasis on exploring processes that allow for community participation in the planning of both services and strategies for health (Laughlin & Black, 1995). In addition, the philosophy of the World Health Organisation *Health for All* (2000) has led to further interest in participatory community projects, i.e. projects that aim for a 'bottom up' approach exploring local issues from working with and within communities (see also Ong & Humphris, 1994).

This chapter will explore ways in which reflexivity facilitated an exploration of identity and (dis-)empowerment throughout the research process. Drawing on examples from the aforementioned research project we will illustrate the fluidity and the tensions experienced negotiating these issues, and ways in which the use of reflexivity aided the articulation of enriched theoretical understandings.

Interrogating feminist presuppositions: hearing young men's voices

The Sheffield Young People's Sexual Health Project emerged from citywide concerns relating to diminishing sexual health, increasing teenage pregnancies and a lack of knowledge on 'invisible' groups (e.g. young people involved in sexual exploitation, young gay men, young carers) among young people in Sheffield. Although excited about the opportunity to participate in such work we quickly became aware of some tensions in our position in relation to the subject area. In particular, our investment in feminist principles which saw patriarchal relations between women and men as problematic (Rich, 1980; Choi, 1994) was challenged. One of the main aims of the project was to provide the women participating with an opportunity to talk about their concerns in a women-friendly environment, and to produce outcomes of benefit to these and other young women. However, as the data collection progressed we became increasingly uncomfortable with discourses on young men as the 'forgotten victims of sexual health services'. Given our feminist commitments, such tensions were practical issues for us that required critical reflection at this pre-research stage. This required us to re-negotiate our positions within planning meetings where we were compelled to listen to, and engage with, debates relating to the experiences of young men from the viewpoint of different agencies contributing to the research. We had to work over a period of time at questioning our resistance to the proposed direction of the research and the challenges this might bring in relation to the content of research tools that were to be employed. There was a need to work towards a greater empathy when engaging with male sexual experiences, a 'head-shift' in acknowledging these as legitimate areas for exploration. We needed to rethink who the research would be 'of use' to, to expand our existing political positions as researchers. As well as the need to shift on a personal level, the need to embody the 'organisational voices' of young men at each level of the research process was highlighted, especially during steering group meetings which oversaw the project.

We feel that our use of reflexivity in the 'pre-researching thinking' stage of the project flagged up our responsibilities to re-visit and re-think our position in relation to how accounts from young men should be addressed as the project proceeded. Initial analysis of the audio-taped interviews reinforced our feminist thinking relating to the ways in which young men can undermine young women's social and sexual positions. However, we also encountered examples of young men attempting to talk and interact in places outside such conventional gender positions. At this stage, reflexivity enabled us to explore and make visible the consequences for young men who attempt to find new spaces to communicate and to deepen their self-understanding. In this way our prior understanding of hegemonic masculinity was unsettled and our knowledge of gender identities considerably enriched. Further analysis moved us towards addressing issues associated with the fragility of, and constraints on, young men's power. Thus, the inclusion of young men's voices provided valuable insights into how young men negotiate their sexual and social identities within certain settings.

In this section we use interview extracts to demonstrate how reflexivity facilitated the loosening of this particular theoretical knot. During the initial stages of the data analysis, the tensions we had experienced during the pre-thinking stage of the research returned as accounts of young men using their power to diminish and regulate young women's sexual identities and practices emerged. For example, during group discussions young women were at times prevented from answering questions or discussing issues due to male interruptions and innuendo:

Peer researcher 1: What is heavy petting?
Sally: Getting warmed up for it (sex), you know.
Adam: See these birds from Newcastle they're not bothered, they'd just say anything.
PR1: [PR continues with research questions] Do you think she's still a virgin?
S: Yes I do.
A: Just dirty lasses …
Mark: Right …
A: Just dirty lasses do everything an' what …
M: Maybe the ones you know.
A: But why the fucking ones that I know?
M: 'Cause you know some right ones.
S: [laughs] I mean these ones that chuck themselves on lighted paper don't they? Not all Geordies are the same … not all them. I mean I'm quite quiet me for a Geordie an' all that.

On other occasions, confrontation by some of the young men was more obvious, signalled by derogatory remarks about the young women's alleged sexual practices:

Peer researcher 1: It says 'if I loved him I would do the things he wants'.
Mary: If I loved him that much – I would yeah.
Cath: And you didn't want him to go [male making noise in the background and another laughing]
Peer researcher 2: Do you think it's a … have you been … has anyone said it to you before … tried to persuade you?
M: No 'cos it's …
Andy: They already get it.
Bob: Yeah [laughter].

Yet as the analysis continued these tensions were further contextualised when we became aware of the complex and multiple ways in which young men were disempowered. For example, it emerged that, unlike the women participating in the research who seemed to have access to a language to describe their experiences (and, on occasion, resist attempts to regulate these), the majority of these young men lacked a language or space to challenge powerful notions of what men are like. Throughout the transcripts some young men talked about pressures not to show feelings, of sexual prowess as one of the main ways to obtain social status and, as the following extract illustrates, the difficulties in challenging how men *should* behave:

Research Development worker: What do you think it'd be ... do you think lads are they more likely to [pick on someone for being a virgin]?
Ant: I don't because emm ...
Nick: Yeah actually ... I think they're more actually ... because emm ... they can ... could be a woman in the sense of questioning the man's emm ... manliness if you know what I mean....
A: Yeah 'cos....
N: Man's reputation will be questioned more of a woman emm ... yeah ... especially ... emm when I were at school I saw people getting the mike taken ... but by women more than men actually emm ... than anything else because they can get away with it though ... men you know would ... when they argue they fight you know ... there's not many men out there that would turn round an' hit women....
Oscar: They still do though....
N: Yeah I know but....
O: An' I think it's sick myself.
N: That's one way of lookin' at it.
RD: What?
O: Blokes hittin' women, I think it's sick....
N: I think it's sick anybody hittin' anybody whether it's a bloke or a woman anyway.
O: Oh if a bloke deserves a good beatin' then that bloke's gonna get a good beatin'.

Our understanding of a degree of precariousness associated with young men's negotiation of their masculinity is illustrated further in the next extract, where participants attempted to explore their ideas and experiences of relationships. For example, in an all-male discussion group, Carlos tries to challenge the idea that men do not have feelings for the women with whom they are involved in relationships, but is immediately mocked by his peers. Indeed, in order to regain his credibility as a 'real' man, Carlos deflects the ridicule by mocking another young man in the group for, ironically, showing his feelings for a girl he had met on holiday:

Carlos: You can have feelin's [last word said very quietly].
Peer researcher 1: Yeah what?
C: Feelin's [laughter from the other young men in the group] ... You can....
PR1: Go on with what you're sayin' [laughter continues from the other young men in the group].
C: [To one of the men in the group] I don't know what you're laughin' at 'cos you had loads of feelin's for that lass on holiday [loud laughter from males in the group].
Chas: You got it wrong [cheering and jeering from the males in the group].

Owen: 'Jerry, Jerry, Jerry' [chanting à la 'Jerry Springer Show', indicating raised tension and humour].

Even though this additional information complicated the picture of how young men are positioned, we experienced tension about what to do with this knowledge. As 'feminist' social researchers we were concerned about simply reproducing a 'men as victims' discourse, since, as males, they still have access to considerable social power, as demonstrated by the first and second extracts above (see Gough & Peace, 2000). At this stage then, reflexivity provided us with the space to explore and discuss the ways in which our political positions could potentially influence the research and how we could place this awareness both theoretically and in terms of policy implications. On the one hand, we were reassured by the dominant picture of young people's worlds presented by the participants, as this strengthens existing feminist writing on gender and sexuality as key sites for identity (Vance, 1984; Holland *et al.*, 1990; Lees, 1993; McFadden, 1995). The recent backlash against 'feminist' agendas and objectives (Faludi, 1992; Gough, 1998) and wider social discourses that propose that gender equality has been achieved are, we hope, undermined by the current analysis. On the other hand, the analysis of the talk of some of the young men participating in this project, and the ways they used language to achieve status in their interactions with other young men, enabled more complex understandings of the fluidity of power and gender in structuring social relations (Foucault, 1978) and the fragility and defensive nature of hegemonic masculinity (Frosh, 1993). A key tenet of feminist work – the understanding that the personal is political – enabled us to suggest strategies relating to the importance of grounding policy and service provision for young men in ways that would enable them to become aware of, and make 'choices' around, what we perceived as largely naturalised (and consequently invisible) constructions of hegemonic masculinity (Connell, 1995). In the interim and final reports on the project we suggested that a key aspect of such work would focus on the emotional and social costs associated with unproblematically accepting or privileging understandings of masculinity that obscure the emotional and social obstacles that young men face negotiating their sexual and social identities within a world structured by diverse and often contradictory needs and desires.

Resisting and re-working power and expertise within the research matrix

Reflexivity provided an invaluable platform for exploring power relations and 'expertise' throughout the duration of the two projects. The importance of these issues cannot be overstated given the young-person-centred ethos of the project. During the research project there were instances of the young people clearly feeling confident around their roles and expertise. For example, at the end of the first phase the peer researchers felt sufficiently equipped to comment critically on the data obtained from the questionnaires, even questioning the supposed expertise of the university researchers ('they should have done it better') and imagining how they (the peer researchers) might improve the study. Listening to such feedback produced initial feelings of annoyance for us – we considered the young people's comments to be overly critical, and quite cheeky! There was also a sense that the research and development workers failed to make any attempt to explain the presentation of the findings, a task that we perceived to be an integral part of their role.

However, such instances were invaluable in challenging our thinking around what constitutes collaborative research. Despite our aim to diminish the power differentials which dog traditional research approaches, we realised that we had overlooked some central issues within the wider research matrix involving young people as users of power. This new awareness and the further use of reflexive practices enabled those involved in the research to identify and communicate practical and emotional concerns resulting from the complex and shifting power relations structuring the project. Such experiences illustrate Brinton-Lyke's (1997) insight that 'collaboration and trust do not negate power differentials; rather they create a bond between two active subjects who must then negotiate the power differential between them as they encounter it.'

The initial phase of the research involved the construction of a young people's questionnaire on sexual health, experiences and obstacles to using service provision. During the designing of this first research tool for the project, reflexivity functioned as an invaluable tool for deconstructing and challenging perceptions of the research consultants as 'the experts' in relation to the methodology. As Sandelowski (1998, p.30) states, 'new modes of participatory research have complicated the role of expert and the idea of expertise.' Reflexive analysis of the research process at this stage enabled both the research and development workers and us (the university-based researchers) to engage with power inequalities as dynamic processes shaping the research – much in the way that two football teams compete for possession of the ball (expertise).

This initial phase ran for a four-month period, with the research and development workers establishing contact with available young people in their host agencies and attempting to integrate diverse development and training needs. In the training that we delivered, it was emphasised to the research and development workers that they were the experts in relation to their knowledge of the groups of young people, as well as the pace at which the two parallel processes should run. Our role was defined as attempting to meet the identified research needs of the research and development workers and the young people. As such, we felt that this approach allowed us to address and re-work notions of 'the expert' embedded in many traditional research relationships.

The two versions of the questionnaires constructed by the research and development workers and the groups of young people made visible our expectations at this stage of the process. Firstly, the questionnaires were not what we had expected. For example, items relating to sexual health omitted what we considered to be significant dimensions, such as avoiding pregnancy and sexually transmitted diseases, being confident enough to use services and being able to resist unwanted attention. In addition, differences in the style and content of the questionnaires led us to question whether the understandings of why and how the research would progress were accessible to the young people.

At this stage we felt we needed to actively reflect on the ways in which we had conducted the training sessions with the research and development workers. Had we been unclear about the objectives of this phase and the research philosophy underpinning the project? Why were we angry and disappointed with the outcome. How should we deal with this? This involved us questioning our assumptions about what we would have liked the questionnaire to contain and whether these expectations were realistic. We looked at how our expectations were shaped by our own research agendas (for example, our desire to pursue questions about sexuality) and also by our current jobs where we predominately deal with the work of third-level university students who receive training on research methods. Attempting to place ourselves in the position of the young people, the majority of whom were novice researchers, proved illuminating.

In respect of the research and development workers, the process was more anxiety-provoking. Tracking back through prior research meetings in an attempt to clarify the main issues regarding the research was a time-consuming and frustrating process. During this process we found ourselves imagining how we would have conducted the research – and sometimes fantasising about the control and fulfilment that doing it ourselves would have offered. We reflected, however, that to develop the questionnaire from its original state would be to undermine the collaborative flavour of the research contract. The decision was therefore made, despite time pressures, to extend this phase and ask the research and development workers to take time to reflect on our comments and how they felt about our proposed changes in the timetabling of the project and their work with the young people.

At this juncture, communication with the research and development workers became fraught, with a hotchpotch of issues emerging, including their time pressures, their established relations with their groups and their faith in us as trainers and so-called research experts. Boundaries with the research and development workers relating to *their* roles as experts were tested. Increasingly, as a result of their anxieties and deteriorating confidence in us, they sought the safety that came with re-positioning us as the experts. With this came accusations that we should have maintained a tighter hold on the research process and highlighted issues at an earlier stage. The need for us to re-negotiate their position as the experts made us aware that the research and development workers were using their power to define themselves in a particular way, one that we did not necessarily endorse. Following much deliberation, we agreed to adopt a more visible role in the research process.

Such reflections allowed the researchers and the research and development workers to explore areas of awareness that otherwise may have been absent from the experience of conducting participatory research. We had assumed that we could re-negotiate understandings of where expertise lies. However, the process made us aware of obstacles that the researcher can face in attempting to deconstruct the discourse of expertise that surrounds social researchers, despite their best intentions. In addition, critical analysis of the processes at this stage in the research forced us to make transparent decisions and justify our decision-making processes.

Reflexivity: problems and prospects

So far this chapter has illustrated the ways in which reflexivity provided an invaluable tool for exploring identities within the research matrix, generating insight into knotty and fluid power dynamics, as well as providing new foundations on which to think and develop theoretical parameters underpinning the research project. In this final section we explore the use of reflexivity in the concluding phase of the project, in particular the ways in which our thinking on, and experience of, identity and (dis)empowerment required making visible the emotional dynamics within the research matrix. In using reflexivity to confront such issues within the project we find ourselves encountering outstanding questions and feel unable to offer a neatly packaged conclusion.

Although the almost constant need to negotiate positions throughout the projects was at times experienced as difficult and frustrating, it was also stimulating and strengthened a sense of involvement among the research team. In general, using reflexivity consolidated awareness that 'collective work is messy and that researchers doing this type of work need to be open to negotiating various positions within the research matrix, including those of 'organiser, educator and researcher' (McGuire, 1993, p.15). This point was illustrated in the latter phase of the project, when changes in staff shifted the dynamic within the research matrix. The appointment of a senior manager to the project, and the subsequent attempt at an organisational or bureaucratic solution to the problem of 'messiness', initially seemed a useful progression.

In hindsight, this new culture impacted significantly on responsibility and power dynamics within the research matrix. Firstly, there was an increasing centralisation of communication that resulted in less discussion within the matrix about roles and responsibilities, and a greater focus on communicating through the senior manager. Secondly, what emerges from our diaries is a sense of no longer being in partnership in quite the same way. The relationship between us and the other members of the team shifted into a servicing agreement in terms of the university and the project. For us, the focus of the project seemed to move from one centred on involving young people in community-based research to getting the job done within the time limit.

Yet, although our earlier research memos clearly describe struggles with this 'messiness', one important lesson we learned was the need to find creative ways to live with the complexity, rather than attempt to solve it. For us, reflexivity provided a foundation upon which the fluidity of roles, the negotiation of power and preserving the dynamic could be framed.

Both of us were attracted to the project as an opportunity to explore the re-working of power within the research relationship, to involve young people actively in the production of knowledge, and to work in partnership with participants more effectively than is possible in traditional research projects. For us, key markers of the project's success were illustrations of empowerment among the young people. In the latter stage of the project, reflexivity provided a space to deconstruct the issue of empowerment and the emotional concerns we shared regarding the extent to which the young people had experienced the process as an empowering one. There are some examples from the project where the young people's identities shift to include the role of researchers and where they define themselves as central to the project. For example, during the process of collecting the survey data for the sexual health project, some of the young people talked about feeling important and 'famous' within their own schools.

From a research point of view, the time factor (analysis was carried out after the official end of the project) meant that young people were excluded from the analysis process. Consequently, the researchers' voices remained somewhat hidden yet powerful within the analysis and writing-up of the qualitative data. This was not what we had originally envisaged when writing the research proposal. For us as researchers, this presented some questions relating to the central aims of working in partnership with young people, and giving visibility to their views. Indeed, this issue was brought home further during the allocation of resources in the final phase of the project. A major consideration for the research team throughout the young people's eighteen-month involvement with this project was that their efforts were recognised and rewarded. In phase one of the project, in order to facilitate group development and recognise the hard work the young people had put into constructing the questionnaire, a weekend trip was organised. Both groups of young people enjoyed this experience and spoke about it with pleasure, indeed one group affectionately named the location 'Skeggy Vegas'. Following this success there was a commitment to take both groups away again towards the end of the project. However, this did not happen. The decision against it was taken in a management meeting with no consultation with the young people or researchers. During the data collection period for the second phase of the project, this issue was revisited during one of the group interviews:

Steven: We're not going on residential anymore.

Carl: Your residential has been cancelled ain't it?

S: Yeah.

Paul: Yeah.

C: 'Cos of that stupid . . . go off sick.

S: Who J?

C: Yeah that woman.

Andrew: No not her, we were told there's a woman who's gone off sick . . . yeah L . . . so they've gotta pay her wages whilst she's off sick as well as pay. . . .

P: [to worker] Can you come with us . . . so we can go on a residential?

C: There ain't enough money you dumb bastard.

P: There is enough money.

Chris: J said there was enough money.

C: There isn't enough money because they've to pay who's off sick.

Worker: Yes . . . so basically we've got to pay her wage whilst she's off sick and then we've got to pay other people to take her place; anyway so it's, it's costing a lot of money.

P: So that's why we're not going on the residential.

In this extract the young people are attempting to present the story they had been given about why the weekend away was cancelled, and the worker provides some input into the explanation which reflected an organisational perspective. Yet for us there is a degree of emotion not addressed in this interaction as the young people reflect on their sense of how this decision was presented to them (as a *fait accompli*) – their sense of loss about the lack of a final residential and their relatively lower status in the allocation and prioritising of resources. From our position, experiencing this interaction after the project has finished, there is discomfort and frustration relating to what we mean when we talk about empowering young people, and we are currently using reflexivity to explore the limitations of this kind of research process. At present, we do not have any neatly packaged answers to this question. Indeed, reflecting on our experiences has generated further questions about this kind of research project. Here are just three of them:

- To what extent is it possible – and fruitful – to document tensions relating to identity and (dis)empowerment?
- Who is empowered in/by participatory research?
- What type of evidence should researchers use to evaluate such research processes?

References

Balcazar, F.E., Keys, C.B., Kaplan, D.L. & Suarez-Balcazar (1998) Participatory action research and people with disabilities: principles and challenges. *Canadian Journal of Rehabilitation*, **12**(2), 1005–112.

Banister, P., Burman., E., Parker, I., Taylor, M. & Tindall, C. (1994) *Qualitative Methods in Psychology: A Research Guide*. Open University Press, Buckingham.

Brinton-Lykes, M.B. (1997) Activist participatory research among the Maya of Guatamala: constructing meanings from situated knowledge. *Journal of Social Issues*, **53**(4), 725–46.

Choi, P.Y.L. (1994) Women's raging hormones. In *Female Sexuality: Psychology, Biology and Social Context* (Choi, P.Y.L. & Nicolson, P., eds). Harvester Wheatsheaf, New York.

Connell, R.W. (1995) *Masculinities*. Polity, Cambridge.

Denzin, N.K. & Lincoln, Y. (1994) *Handbook of Qualitative Research*. Sage Publications, Thousand Oaks, CA.

Faludi, S. (1992) *Backlash: The Undeclared War Against Women*. Chatto & Windus, London.

Foucault, M. (1978) *The History of Sexuality: An Introduction*. Penguin Press, London.

Frosh, S. (1993) The seeds of male sexuality. In *Psychological Perspectives on Sexual Problems* (Ussher, J. & Baker, C., eds). Routledge, London.

Gough, B. (1998) Men and the discursive reproduction of sexism: repertoires of difference and equality. *Feminism & Psychology*, **8**(1), 25–49.

Gough, B. (1999) 'Subject positions within discourse analysis: some reflexive dilemmas'. Paper given at *International Human Science Research Conference*, Sheffield Hallam Univeristy, July.

Gough, B. & Peace, P. (2000) Reconstructing gender in the 1990s: men as victims. *Gender & Education*, **12**(3), 385–99.

Holland, J., Ramazanoglu, C. & Scott, S. (1990) *Sex, Risk, Danger: AIDS Education Policy and Young Women's Sexuality*. The Tufnell Press, London.

Laughlin, S. & Black, D. (1995) *Poverty and Health Tools for Change*. A Public Health Trust Project. Public Health Alliance, Birmingham.

Lees, S. (1993) *Sugar and Spice: Sexuality and Adolescent Girls*. Penguin, London.

McFadden, M. (1995) *Female Sexuality in the Second Decade of AIDS*. PhD thesis, The Queen's University, Belfast.

McGuire, P. (1993) Challenges, contradictions and celebrations: attempting participatory research as a doctoral student. In *Voices of Change: Participatory Research in the United States and Canada* (Park, P., Brydon-Miller, M., Hall, B. & Jackson, T., eds). Bergin & Garvey, Westport.

Ong, B.N. & Humphris, G. (1994) Prioritizing needs with communities. In: *Researching the People's Health* (Popay, J. & Williams, G., eds). Routledge, London.

Reason, P. (ed.) (1988) *Human Inquiry in Action*. Sage Publications, London.

Rich, A. (1980) Compulsory heterosexuality and lesbian existence. *Signs*, **5**(4), 631–60.

Sandelowski, M. (1998) The call to experts in qualitative research. *Research in Nursing and Health*, **21**(5), 467–71.

Sannchez, R.D. & Juarez, M.P. (1995) Community based health research & advocacy on health among poor women in Davao City, Philippines. *Reproductive Health Matters*, 5, 89–94.

Seale, C. (1999) *The Quality of Qualitative Research*. Sage Publications, London.

Vance, C. (1984) *Pleasure and Danger: Exploring Female Sexuality*. Routledge, London.

Wetherell, M. & Maybin, J. (1996) The distributed self: a social constructionist perspective. In *Understanding The Self* (Stevens, R., ed.). Sage/Open University Press, London.

Wilkinson, S. (1988) The role of reflexivity in feminist psychology. *Women's Studies International Forum*, 11, 493–502.

CHAPTER 16

Holding up the mirror to widen the view: multiple subjectivities in the reflexive team

Christine A. Barry

Positioning the self: author's story

I have been an academic researcher for eleven years and am currently based at Brunel University. I draw on the disciplines of anthropology, sociology and psychology in my research on health, illness, health care and healing. I studied psychology at Birkbeck College and have worked on a sociological ethnographic study of the use of the internet amongst academics, a psychological study of stress and depression in cancer patients, and a medical sociological study of doctor–patient communication in general practice. I am currently conducting an anthropological ethnographic comparative study of the culture of alternative medicine inside and outside the National Health Service for my doctorate. As a constructivist who believes in the multiple perspectives of both participants and researchers, I agree with Charlotte Aull Davies that the products of research are affected by the personnel involved and the process of doing research. She suggests that the personal history of researchers, their disciplinary background, and the socio-cultural circumstances in which they have worked have profound effects on what they study, how they study it and how they interpret their data (Davies, 1999). I believe that 'the specificity and individuality of the observer are ever present and must therefore be acknowledged, explored and put to creative use' (Okely, 1996, p.28). The position I take is one of the need for continual reflexivity throughout the research process and the need for the researcher(s) to be fully present in the published accounts of research.

I think doing reflexivity alone is difficult and should always be aided by the input of academic colleagues and supervisors. Where research is done as a team activity the opportunities for critical reflexivity are multiplied. Where research is multidisciplinary, as in the project team I write about here, the opportunities for a deep and rich reflexive insight are increased. The tensions in this process may also be greater.

I have just completed an anthropological ethnographic comparative study of the culture of alternative medicine inside and outside the National Health Service for my doctorate.

Introduction

'Improving doctor–patient communication about prescribing' is an ongoing project I have been involved with since 1996. For the first three years I worked as a research fellow in this multi-disciplinary collaborative project. The team included two sociologists, Nicky Britten and Fiona Stevenson; an academic GP, Colin Bradley; and an academic social pharmacist, Nick Barber.

My interest in group processes, interpersonal issues, communication and emotional aspects led me to encourage more openness and reflexivity when I joined the team. Experiences with small-group teaching meant that others in the team were also interested in group processes and so were receptive to my ideas. In some teams the personal anxiety and defensiveness of individuals would not allow this openness to thrive. Delaney and Ames (1993) note that in their team the lead reflexive role was taken on by the anthropologists (interestingly I have now become an anthropologist). Given my own inclination towards reflexivity, I was as interested in analysing the team processes as I was in analysing the processes of patients and their doctors. I was aided in this endeavour by the insights of my good friend David Afia who operated as an impartial critical adviser, drawing on his work on the psychodynamic aspects of organisations.

In order to encourage a climate of group reflexivity I proposed early on to my team that we engage collectively in two specific reflexive tasks: (1) writing and sharing reflexive statements about our own position in the research at intervals through the project and, (2) writing theoretical definitions of key theoretical concepts. In both cases these individual pieces of writing of team members were shared and discussed in regular team meetings, leading to a heightened reflexive awareness in the team and to improved and enriched analysis of data emerging from the project.

Before detailing our reflexive approach I will outline the nature of our project and the research team.

Project background and design

The project is funded by the British government's Department of Health. It is a study of doctor–patient communication about prescribing in general practice. The idea for the research arose out of the paradox that doctors complain about patients 'demanding' prescriptions while patients would prefer their general practitioners to prescribe less and communicate more. The aim of phase I, a two-year qualitative study (1996–98), was to explore the reasons for this paradox and then to use the information gained to design and evaluate educational interventions (phase II 1998–2002). In this paper I concentrate on the activities of the team during phase I, when I was a full-time research fellow on the project.

Phase I consisted of case studies with 65 patients in 20 practices. This involved selecting a surgery day with each of 20 general practitioners, contacting patients once they had made an appointment and interviewing them at home (or, in the case of emergency patients, interviewing them in the surgery before their consultation). The doctors audiotaped the consultations and were interviewed later about their perceptions of the consultation. The patients were interviewed at home a week later about their views and their subsequent actions. The interviews were semi-structured but patients were encouraged to talk about their own concerns within this structure. The aim of this design was to link expectations and perceptions of patients and doctors about a specific consultation to what actually happened in the consultation, and also to what patients did with their medicines afterwards.

The substantive findings of the project have been published elsewhere (Bradley *et al.*, 1999; Stevenson *et al.*, 1999; Barry *et al.*, 2000; Britten *et al.*, 2000; Barry *et al.*, 2001; Stevenson *et al.*, 2002). More detail on the methodology can be found in Stevenson *et al.* (2000) and Barry (2002).

Reflexive tasks to aid the process of awareness and communication

Geography had a big impact on the project. Being located in three, later four, sites meant that the team missed out on informal and formal face-to-face opportunities for communication. To counteract this we met as a team for a whole day every six weeks to discuss the project (once a month for the first few months). This provided a valuable arena for reflexive discussions.

Our team's reflexive approach involved raising awareness of the orientation of team members and then an iterative process of communication and negotiation to come to a team consensus. This process helped us to build a productive team. As a team we engaged in two group reflexive writing projects. We also engaged in writing individual reflexive diaries, fieldnotes and memos and in discussing the processes and structures of the team (all these activities were interlinked). In the first of the specific group projects we used a reflexive account of *our individual orientation* and the second comprised an exercise around *definitions of key theoretical concepts*. Both exercises were conducted towards the start of the project and subsequently once a year throughout the life of the project. All the documents generated by this process were circulated to the team and discussed as a group.

In this section I give examples of how the knowledge arising from these exercises impacted on the research project. I firstly detail the two methods (see Boxes 16.1 and 16.2) and give examples of reflexive data produced by our group during the two exercises. I then go on to show how these examples came to be important in the development of the project. To do this I present the details of one specific analytic discussion of substantive data: 'the seaweed incident' (see Box 16.3).

Accounting for individual orientations

Box 16.1 Team reflexive accounts – the first task

At our first full team meeting, I bring the issue of team functioning into the spotlight by circulating a paper on qualitative teaming (Liggett *et al.*, 1994), and suggest that we each write and share reflexive position statements structured around the following orienting questions:

- In what way might my experience colour my participation in the project?
- What experience have I had with qualitative research?
- What is my orientation to qualitative research?
- What results do I expect to come out of this project?
- What theoretical lens do I favour to apply to the results?
- What is my stake in the research? What do I hope to get out of it?
- What are my fears?

Despite feeling some uncertainty, the team agree to write their position statements, in part because we all agree with the philosophy behind it and in part because we want to maintain group unity at this early stage. With hindsight, it was possibly too early in the life of the team to do this – it caused some anxiety. It might have been better to let the team engage in some bonding and gain confidence and trust in each other before embarking on this type of exercise. As Erickson and Stull (1998) point out, a team needs to undergo a period of team bonding where social activities such as shared meals can be very important.

The exercise proves to be a shortcut to an increased understanding of our own and each other's positions and in itself precipitates team bonding. Being prepared to be honest and open about our biases, hopes and fears encourages a climate of openness. It also fosters increased commitment to the team. Our being prepared to reveal vulnerabilities and areas in which we are less confident draws us closer to each other and develops trust. We learn more about each other in a condensed space of time than we might have ever achieved through the life of the project, without this intervention. We learn details of each other's family culture with relation to health and illness, personal experiences of health care and career trajectories.

My aim in listing orienting questions is to help the members of the team less used to reflexive writing. However, this unwittingly reveals my own conception of the important issues for reflexive thinking, and the others take issue. In the event, each of us answers the questions we can relate to, but we also write about other issues we feel are important. In this way the team engages in the task with commitment and enthusiasm and gains ownership of what was initially my strategy.

The team evolved over a couple of years from the initial proposal development phase in which the three project directors (Nick, Colin and Nicky) were involved, to incorporating myself and Fiona as research fellows when funding was obtained. Prior to our arrival the team of three project directors were able to conform to a collegial structure: all were of similar status and age, all had equal responsibilities with regard to the project, and all had goals in common. With the addition of us two researchers, there was an inevitable shift towards greater hierarchy. This was partly linked to the different agendas and goals of the project leaders and researchers (see Wakeford, 1985) but also to the nature of the split in workload. As full-time researchers we were responsible for participant recruitment, fieldwork, and the lengthy business of qualitative data analysis. The main concerns for the three senior members were to ensure we kept to the remit of our funders regarding timeframe and budget, and were producing our promised output. This led to a two-tier team structure. (See Erickson & Stull, 1998 for a discussion of the double team approach.) Table 16.1 summarises the roles of the personnel in the project.

Table 16.1　Team personnel and roles in phase 1 of the project.

Name	Nicky	Nick	Colin	Christine	Fiona
Discipline	Sociology	Pharmacy	General practice	Psychology	Sociology
Position	Senior Lecturer	Professor	Professor	Research Fellow	Research Fellow
Project planning	•	•	•		
Obtaining funding	•	•	•		
Questionnaire design				•	•
Fieldwork				•	•
Coding and analysis	•			•	•
Writing	•	•	•	•	•

The reflexive writing process helped the team strive to reduce this hierarchical element and maintain as collegial an approach as possible. The fact that all five of us were prepared to write openly about our hidden agendas, interests and fears about the project, and to spend time reading and reflecting on the standpoints of others, fostered democracy and friendship within the team. This early experience helped to produce a climate of fairness where all members have an equal right to express an opinion about the research in meetings and to be taken seriously.

Much of the information we learned through this early exercise (Box 16.1) helped to smooth the project along later on. For example, at this early stage it was easy to delineate individuals' main area of interest in the data, and to see that overlaps of interest were less common than we had imagined, reducing fears that our subsequent publications might compete with each other. There seemed to be enough diversity for us all to be able to pursue our own particular interests in the data. Gaining this awareness early in the project enabled us to discuss our viewpoints in more detail and to move towards common ground. We formed alliances to plan particular papers and avoid conflict that might have occurred had these issues arisen later, during the pressurised writing-up period.

Theoretical reflexivity

The discovery of our diversity also helped develop and strengthen the rigour of our theoretical thinking. If we had all shared the same views there might have been a lack of self-questioning: we might have become lazy in our thinking and failed to broaden our individual thinking. For example, our positions on the central issue of prescribing differed markedly. In our written reflexive accounts we reported quite different personal orientations to medicine. Fiona, Nicky and myself all admitted to being wary of medication, citing family influences, bad side-effect experiences and direct experience of working in the pharmaceutical industry. However, Nick, with experience as a practising hospital pharmacist, was much more positive about medication. He wrote that he would much prefer to take a drug than suffer with a headache. He, too, cited family experiences as relevant: his mother had always been ready to produce remedies to cure ailments. Colin's perspective as a GP revealed an implicit recognition of the potential harm of drugs, reported very much from the prescriber end of the process. He was the only member of the team not to write about his experiences as a patient in his reflexive account. We discovered, then, our quite different views of medication – views rooted in family background and career histories. This helped us, during the analysis stage, to focus more closely than we might otherwise have done on the views of both doctors and patients regarding medication.

As well as marking out our different territories, the written accounts revealed more overlap in our world views than we expected. This calmed our worries about possible incompatibilities. As is well known, 'the team that speaks with more than one voice is doomed' (Gow, 1991, p. 12). As new members of the team, Fiona and I were comforted to discover that neither the GP nor the pharmacist were uncritical supporters of the biomedical model. Instead, there was consensus within the team on the importance of qualitative methods. We found we all believed in a more holistic or biopsychosocial model of medicine and on the need for increased patient autonomy in health care – beliefs and values which would have taken much longer to surface without this reflexive intervention.

In our reflexive discussions it emerged that the three of us who were social scientists focused more than the two health professionals on our favoured theoretical approach – perhaps reflecting different levels of theoretical input in the training within the different disciplines. We recognised that, by the stage of writing-up, we needed to know more about our theoretical underpinnings in order to present a coherent argument and be able to answer critical questions about our methods. Theory would also become an important issue in phase II of the project: designing our educational intervention. Uppermost in our minds was the need to improve the rigour and the quality of our end product. This is particularly important in the medical research arena where qualitative research is not well-understood and is treated with some mistrust. For the three qualitative researchers in the team, we saw the project as an opportunity to fly the flag for qualitative research and convert a few 'non-believers' through a systematic and rigorous approach.

Box 16.2 Team theoretical definitions – the second task

A couple of months into the project, I suggest a second reflexive task to direct our attention to key theoretical issues: each of us should write definitions of the topics we see as representing the central conceptual issues at the heart of the project looking at doctor–patient communication about prescribing. The key theoretical concepts/issues we focus on are:

- Models of illness and health
- Optimum patient care (in general practice)
- Good communication
- The function of language
- Power in GP–patient relationships
- The role of medicine in society
- Informed consent
- Concordance (in place of compliance)
- Education

We aim to ground ourselves in the theory from the literature, recognising the common and dangerous trap of atheoretical qualitative research in health care (Silverman, 1998), and to make sure we all mean the same thing when we use various theoretical terms.

The exercise described in Box 16.2 changed our thinking as individuals. Colin reported that being asked to examine concepts such as models of illness, optimum patient care, and the role of medicines changed his whole slant on the project and also on his own practice as a GP. This process intensified through the period of analysis and further conceptual discussion. He reported a growing understanding that his patients were not just concerned about medicines and might want other things from him as a GP (for example, recognition of their problems as individual human beings). This was felt to be a significant outcome for the project: the changes in thinking reported by our own team GP gave us hope for changing the views of other doctors in phase II of the project.

Differences, even subtle ones, emerging from our theoretical definitions turned out to be important. For example, while our reflexive accounts suggested that we were all advocating greater patient autonomy, our attempts to root our positions in the existing literature revealed several differences. This led us to think more conceptually about our data and gave us a more grounded theoretical base for the project. For example, in her theoretical definition Nicky identified patient autonomy as a key defining factor in the doctor–patient relationship, with the optimum relationship being one of maximum achievable equality. She wrote:

'I think good communication involves: (1) both parties understanding the other's agenda without making too many untested assumptions and (2) a subsequent negotiation about what is to be done ... I think the notion of informed consent is very tricky, because it is unlikely that the lay person will ever have the same level of understanding ... perhaps the crux of the issue (informed consent) is to find out what it is the patient wants to know and what is their frame of reference, so that the explanation / information offered is appropriate for that individual at that time and in that situation.'

Nick, however, was less insistent on the need for patient autonomy. He believed it all depended on the degree to which an individual patient desired autonomy and also on their need to be cared for:

'In most cases, the patient should be treated as an autonomous individual and the doctor should use his/her knowledge to meet their goals, or to refine their goals into feasible ones. It may be that the patient does not want this role ... people who feel ill often revert to being childlike and wanting a nurturing parent; they may just want to be cared for.'

These written statements of theoretical ideas led to a series of forays into the literature.

The 'seaweed incident' – an example

Once the analysis phase had begun, the differences revealed by our reflexive accounts on issues such as patient autonomy became incorporated into the analysis, enriching the interpretations. In analysing the pilot data, we jokingly referred to one particular consultation as the 'seaweed incident' (see Box 16.3).

Our discussions of this consultation showed how our reflexive writings and discussions about patient autonomy had influenced our analytic discussions, enhancing the quality of our interpretations and in turn influencing our ideas about possible communication skills training for phase II. These discussions were recorded in detail. The minutes, prepared after each meeting, were designed not only to record decisions taken and actions required but also to register fresh theoretical insights and themes to incorporate into future analysis.

Box 16.3   Contesting a prescribing communication

Here, we give the patient the pseudonym Jeremy Smythe. He reports to his GP that he is suffering from indigestion.[1] Dr O'Neill suggests referring him to a specialist for a diagnostic endoscopy. During the consultation Jeremy states a preference for avoiding taking drugs. In spite of this Dr O'Neill prescribes an antacid for him to take while waiting for the appointment to come through. As we are particularly interested in communication about prescribing we focus on how the doctor talks about the antacid prescription to Jeremy.

Dr: And what I would do until then . . .

J: Mm.

Dr: . . . is put you on an antacid which is actually just made from seaweed. Okay? It's er you know that jelly-like stuff you get in s . . . when you tread on seaweed?

J: Yeah.

Dr: Well they've made, made it into . . . they've made it into tablets and they've made It into . . .

J: Yeah.

Dr: . . . suspension.

We all saw this piece of communication differently. The differences were sharpest between Nick, the pharmacist, and Nicky, the medical sociologist. Nick considered Dr O'Neill's strategy to be user-friendly, appropriate and positive communication about prescribing – an example which he thought we could use as good practice in the training of other doctors. Nicky, however, saw this presentation as misleading, unnecessarily manipulative, and a poor strategy for communication about prescribing. This led to a heated discussion centred on the degree to which Dr O'Neill was seen as manipulative in talking about the drug in terms of a harmless ingredient, seaweed.

In Nick's view, Jeremy had expressed a desire for symptom relief and so it was appropriate for Dr O'Neill, in his role as carer, to encourage Jeremy to take suitable medication. Nick viewed the doctor's use of the seaweed description as an attempt to use lay beliefs and to talk in the voice of the life world (as distinct from the voice of medicine) (Mishler, 1984).[2]

Nicky, however, focused on Dr O'Neill's failure to offer the patient any choice and his attempt to 'sell' the drug to the patient. She saw him as attempting to influence Jeremy in a paternalistic manner and felt that the description of the

---

[1] Jeremy's case is analysed at greater length in Barry *et al.* (2001).

[2] See Barry *et al.* (2001) for an analysis based on Mishler's concepts of the voices of medicine and of the life world.

antacid as 'just made from seaweed' was an attempt to present the drug as natural, and therefore completely harmless. She would have preferred more discussion in the consultation to ascertain whether the patient's priority was symptom relief or concern about diagnosis. If it had been ascertained that the patient definitely did want to take a drug, which did not seem to be the case here, she would have preferred Dr O'Neill to have presented the drug in a more balanced light.

This debate exposed the difficulty, if we were all going to interpret the data so differently, of pinpointing good practice in our analysis. This became an important issue in our continuing analysis of the phase I data and in our designs for doctor education in phase II. How could we do either if we could not understand each other's viewpoint? Without the reflexive exercises we might have reached a deadlock with no one willing to give ground on which was the 'right' interpretation. However, having read and discussed our reflexive writings it was easier for us to understand and work with the differences of opinion. We could all see where the various team members were coming from. Our different interpretations of the data reflected different theoretical definitions of patient care and different orientations to medicines. This took some of the heat out of the debate.

While the seaweed incident might seem like a trivial example, it proved to be quite pivotal. A number of consequences followed from our discussions and the related reflexive awareness of our positions:

- Realising that our individual interpretations were very much grounded in our prior beliefs and preferred models made it important to develop some criteria external to the individual researcher's assessment in order to judge whether or not a consultation technique was successful. We compiled a number of more 'objective' outcome measures to judge effectiveness of communication. For example, did the communication leave patients with misunderstandings about their drugs? Did the patients subsequently cash the prescriptions they were given?
- We widened the analysis to incorporate doctors' views of medicines. We wanted to see if we could spot any correlation between this and their consulting communication styles. This revealed that both doctors' and patients' views of medicines are important aspects determining behaviour.
- We grasped the importance of reaching a group consensus on our preferred model of communicating about drugs if we were to develop an educational model. This necessitated many more discussions.
- We realised that our existing conceptions of the models of medicine were insufficiently developed or robust to enable us to reach a consensus or to develop a useful model for the doctors in our education phase. This led us back to the literature and helped us develop our conceptions of autonomy by grounding them in the literature on patient-centredness (Stewart *et al.*,1995) and shared decision making (Charles *et al.*, 1997; Coulter, 1997).

Had we not been aware of each other's starting positions we might have foundered, unable to see why we were unable to agree, assuming that when using a term like 'patient autonomy' we all meant the same thing. Knowledge about our differences gave us a more solid base for exploring ideas. The seaweed story was just one example where the knowledge and insight gained from the reflexive accounts helped us negotiate and communicate better. Our more developed ideas about models of patient care fed into our analysis, enabled us to come to a consensus, and helped us revise our proposals to the Department of Health for phase II.

Discussion

We believe that team reflexivity intensifies the benefits and minimises the pitfalls of the team approach. Through sharing common ground, enabling multiple voices to emerge and developing a productive dialectic, we believe we improved our conceptual thinking, capitalised on our multiple disciplines, and improved the rigour and quality of our research.

Communicating and negotiating our differences has broadened our views and increased the rigour of our theoretical thinking. Nothing is taken for granted: positions have to be thought through and weak arguments exposed. Our differences have also stopped us from becoming too cosy or complacent. Each of us has had to think hard to justify our ideas and be willing to shift ground. Had these differences surfaced later, at the writing-up stage, they would almost inevitably have raised tensions and increased the likelihood that individual power would have prevailed over rational argument.

There are multiple voices in this area of applied health care research: the patient, the doctor, the pharmacist, the academic, the educator. Many research projects speak with only one of these voices. However, once findings are published they become the property of *all voices*. Patient-centred research, for example, has to take on the critics from the worlds of biomedicine. The strength of multidisciplinary reflexivity is that the multiple voices exist *within*. Using reflexivity to uncover the different agendas of each team member helps us to avoid biasing the data towards one voice. It also helps us, to some extent, to predict and deal with potential criticism before publication.

Minimising mis-communication within our own team seems particularly important on a project studying communication. Reflexivity has helped us to see our team meetings as a metaphor for the meetings between doctors and patients. If optimum patient care involves patients being encouraged to communicate their agendas and doctors to communicate alternatives and uncertainties, then we should practise what we preach. In examining our team's own communication problems we have gained more insight into doctor–patient communication. In spite of our reflexive openness as a team we still experience our fair share of poor communication and misunderstanding. Investigating the reasons for this has helped us to understand why such misunderstandings might also exist in the surgery. Failing to see things through the eyes of the other party, making assumptions without checking back, not allowing the agendas of both parties to emerge, allowing emotions to dictate action: these are some of the concepts we have developed in our analysis of medical consultation (see Barry *et al.*, 2000) and that we have understood experientially from examining our own meetings.

As well as optimising the strengths of the team, this approach helps to minimise the pitfalls and reduces the impact of the academic cult of individualism (Erickson & Stull, 1998). Tendencies towards competitiveness, seeking to appropriate sections of the data, or possessiveness about ideas have been reduced while feelings of team loyalty, consensus and sharing in the ownership of ideas have been strengthened.

Where disputes in the team have emerged, there has been less head-on conflict as people have tried hard to understand others' point of view. For example, the debate over the seaweed incident was settled by everyone accepting that different interpretations resulted from different theoretical standpoints: therefore there was no need for anyone to 'be right'. The only other major dispute we had concerned the way in which the presentation of qualitative data might have to be compromised in order to get published in the *British Medical Journal*. Respect for each other's differing standpoints, and the growing sense of team belonging led us to a successful resolution in accepting each other's different views and working towards a compromise solution. This might not have happened had we been a less cohesive team.

Of course, some problems and tensions persisted. As research fellows trying to deal with day-to-day problems in the field, we sometimes felt insufficiently supported by the project directors. At times, not every team member was seen to be making an equal contribution to the writing process. However, such problems were minimised by the reduced sense, in our team, of 'us and them' divisions. There was a real sense of 'belonging' and of understanding one another. All this was helped by the active adoption of a reflexive approach.

Obviously, this exercise is not being carried out as a randomised controlled trial: we cannot know how we would have worked as a team without the strong element of reflexivity. However, it is interesting to note that we are not experiencing the problems of collaborative writing highlighted by other authors (e.g. Erickson & Stull, 1998). We have so far worked together successfully on twelve papers, a couple of reports and a funding proposal. However it would be fair to say that the writing as a team has been more time-consuming than writing as individuals would have been.

Time is a pitfall mentioned in the literature on team research (e.g. Olesen *et al.*, 1994). For geographical reasons we gave less time to reflexive discussions than we might have liked, yet even meeting once every six weeks made a difference. This was a substantial investment of time over a three-year period; all five members of the team were present at all but one meeting, demonstrating real commitment. Reflecting on the reason for this, we realise that as well as the project, we as individuals are gaining from this process. Over the course of these meetings we have bonded as a team with a common mission, developed our intellectual ideas, broadened our mental boundaries, and developed our inter-personal skills. The time has been well spent.

As a team we have seen the reflexive exercises prove successful in terms of process, project quality and team output. We have improved and refined our methodological approach. We have enriched our analysis and theoretical thinking. We kept to project deadlines, completed fieldwork successfully and produced the required conference presentations and published papers.

Summary

There are three factors about our team that may well have aided its success. Firstly, we had sufficient common ground amongst us at the start. We all share a belief in the qualitative approach, a holistic model of medicine and the need for increased patient participation in decision making. This makes negotiation on lesser points possible. Where teams start from diametrically opposed viewpoints the process of communication and negotiation will be very much harder. Secondly, none of us has a strong personal need or desire to work within a pyramidal hierarchy structure. Not all being based in the same institution, or being dependent on each other for career development, has also reduced the need for hierarchical interaction within our team. Unlike some academics, we are all predisposed to collaborative working and thrive on the social aspects of working with others. A team with a stronger sense of hierarchy might well find the necessary exposure to vulnerability and possibilities for negotiation required by this approach much reduced. Finally, we share a willingness to be open and a preparedness to learn from each other. We seem to have a capacity for airing differences of opinion, being accepting of others' positions and avoiding overt conflict. While we have had some heated discussions, we have retained respect for other opinions, and have ended up laughing over a drink after the day's meeting. These qualities, perhaps, are not to be found in every research team – but the process of reflexivity may help to kindle them.

Acknowledgements

With kind permission from Sage Publications Ltd, this chapter has been reprinted substantially from Barry, C.A., Britten, N., Barber, N., Bradley, C. & Stevenson, F. (1999) Using reflexivity to optimise teamwork in qualitative research. *Qualitative Health Research*, **9**(1), 26–44.

References

Atkinson, J.M. & Heritage, J. (1984) *Structures in Social Action: Studies in Conversation Analysis*. Cambridge University Press, Cambridge.

Barry, C.A., Stevenson, F., Barber, N.D., Bradley, C.P. & Britten, N. (1998) *Doctor–Patient Communication About Prescribing in General Practice: A Qualitative Study*. A report to the Department of Health.

Barry, C.A., Britten, N., Barber, N., Bradley, C. & Stevenson, F. (1999) Using reflexivity to optimise teamwork in qualitative research. *Qualitative Health Research*, **9**(1), 26–44.

Barry, C.A., Bradley, C.P., Britten, N., Stevenson, F.A. & Barber, N. (2000) Patients' unvoiced agendas in general practice consultations: a qualitative study. *British Medical Journal*, 320, 1246–50.

Barry, C.A., Stevenson, F., Britten, N., Barber, N. & Bradley, C. (2001) Giving voice to the lifeworld. More humane, more effective medical care? *Social Science and Medicine*, 53, 487–505.

Barry, C.A. (2002) Multiple realities in a study of medical consultations. *Qualitative Health Research*, **12**(8), 1052–70.

Bradley, C., Crowley, M., Barry, C.A., Stevenson, F.A., Britten, N. & Barber, N. (1999) Patient-centredness and outcomes in primary care. *British Journal of General Practice*, Feb., **149**.

Britten, N., Stevenson, F.A., Barry, C.A., Barber, N. & Bradley, C. (2000) Misunderstanding in prescribing decisions in general practice: a qualitative study. *British Medical Journal*, 320, 484–8.

Charles, C., Gafni, A. & Whelan, T. (1997) Shared decision-making in the medical encounter: what does it mean? (or It takes at least two to tango). *Social Science and Medicine*, **44**(5), 681–92.

Coulter, A. (1997) Partnership with patients: the pros and cons of shared clinical decision-making. *Journal of Health Services Research Policy*, **2**, 112–21.

Davies, C.A. (1999) *Reflexive Ethnography: a Guide to Researching Selves and Others*. Routledge, London.

Delaney, W. & Ames, G. (1993) Integration and exchange in multidisciplinary alcohol research. *Social Science & Medicine*, **44**, 681–92.

Erickson, K.C. & Stull, D.D. (1998) Doing team ethnography: warnings and advice. *Qualitative Research Methods Series*, Volume 42. Sage Publications, Thousand Oaks, CA.

Gow, D.D. (1991) Collaboration in development consulting: stooges, hired guns, or muskateers. *Human Organization*, **50**, 1–15.

Liggett, A.M., Glesne, C.E., Johnston, A.P., Hasazi, S.B. & Schattman, R.A. (1994) Teaming in qualitative research: lessons learned. *Qualitative Studies in Education*, 7(1), 77–88.

Mishler, E.G. (1984) *The Discourse of Medicine: Dialectics of Medical Interviews*. Ablex, New Jersey.

Okely, J. (1996) *Own or Other Culture*. Routledge, London.

Olesen, V., Droes, N., Hatton, D., Chico, N. & Schatzman, L. (1994) Analyzing together:

recollections of a team approach. In *Analyzing Qualitative Data* (Burgess, R.G., ed.). Routledge, London.

Silverman, D. (1998) The quality of qualitative health research: the open-ended interview and its alternatives. *Social Sciences in Health*, 4(2) 104–18.

Stevenson, F., Barry, C.A., Britten, N., Bradley, C.P. & Barber, N.D. (1999) Doctor–patient communication about drugs: the evidence for shared decision making. *Social Science and Medicine*, **50**, 829–40.

Stevenson, F.A., Britten, N., Barry, C.A., Barber, N.D. & Bradley, C.P. (2000) Qualitative methods and prescribing research. *Journal of Clinical Pharmacy and Therapeutics*, **25**(5), 317–24.

Stevenson, F.A., Britten, N., Barry, C.A., Bradley, C.P. & Barber, N. (2002) Perceptions of legitimacy: the influence on medicine taking and prescribing. *Health*, **6**(1), 85–104.

Stewart, M., Brown, J.B., Weston, W.W., McWhinney, I.R., McWilliam, C.L. & Freeman, T.R. (1995) *Patient-Centred Medicine: Transforming the Clinical Method*. Sage Publications, Thousand Oaks, CA.

Wakeford, J. (1985) A Director's Dilemmas. In *Field Methods in the Study of Education* (Burgess, R.G., ed.). Falmer Press, Lewes, East Sussex.

Epilogue

As we have seen, reflexivity can be defined and practised in myriad ways.
Reflexivity can be viewed with suspicion as a distraction from the phenomenon
under scrutiny, or embraced as a valuable means of contextualising knowledge-
making within the research process. Whatever position one takes, most would
agree that reflexivity implies a series of challenges and opportunities for any
qualitative researcher. The final contribution by Katie MacMillan echoes this
point. She adopts a playful and hyper-reflexive writing style in order to interrogate both the notion of reflexivity itself and criticisms directed at reflexive
researchers. Here she draws upon the work of Ashmore (1989) and others to
present a diverting and thought-provoking analysis which blends academic
writing with literary forms such as poetry and dramatic presentation.

CHAPTER 17

The next turn: reflexively analysing reflexive research

Katie MacMillan

Positioning the self: author's story

Katie MacMillan

MacMillan's original biography was invaded by her text 'alters', Scribbler and Sleepstone, who have now heavily edited MacMillan's exaggerated claims of expertise as a reflexive writer. Although she insists on single authorship for her doctoral thesis on hypnosis and poetry, MacMillan's role was overstated. Her long-term interest in therapy has been inspired and guided by Sleepstone, her mentor, and her poems are frequently ghost-written by Scribbler. The reach of MacMillan's current research into the False Memory/Recovered Memory debate (with colleagues at Loughborough University) would undoubtedly be enhanced by the presence of these two experienced (and modest) reflexivists.

Evangeline Scribbler

Although the same has often been said about Sleepstone, Scribbler has also been an accomplished speed boat racer for a number of years. She does not collect railway tickets, phone numbers or umbrellas, and, for the analytical execution performed by Ashmole, she appeared to have tied her shoelaces back to front (they were dark brown) and spoke without a lisp.

Sybil Sleepstone

As well as 'wise' (Meaning of Names, Ethwell's Comprehensive Book of Fortune, 1927), and 'a genius' (MacMillan, 2003), Sleepstone has been fortunate enough to be identified as 'pretentious and evasive' (Editorial Comment, 2002). She is currently piloting a new form of Pretentious Textual Therapy, which will involve using the latest new literary form – that of positioning the self – to insert hidden hypnotic suggestions. Sleepstone expects this new form of therapeutic writing will radicalise social science research within the next few years.

Introduction

The following discussion shows how reflexivity turns analysis upon itself, so that the business of doing research becomes the central topic under investigation. Reflexivity bites, as it were, by drawing attention to the role of the analyst as she constructs her 'data' from research 'subjects' and 'topics.' This radical method of analysis extends the scope of social science research by challenging what is standardly left unchallenged – the assumptions built into traditional data collection and research methodology. Moreover, this reflexive 'next turn' takes another twist on the reflexive spiral. In analysing the process of reflexive research itself I aim to show how reflexivity works, but also how, ironically, the creation of a 'model' of reflexivity will result in a set of prescriptive steps, which will, inevitably, take its method for granted. In order to maintain reflexivity's potential for radical deconstruction, reflexive research should be committed to thorough, ongoing assessment of research practice. This means a lively, engaged reworking of 'rules', reflexive and otherwise, and a dedicated uncertainty for what the object of research might show us, before the method of retelling becomes the story of the event itself.

The central topics of my own research arose from a long-term interest in poetry, my practice at that time as a hypnotherapist, and the serendipitous selection of a doctoral supervisor who turned out to be an expert in reflexive analysis. The supervisor was 'Mr Reflexivity' (MacMillan, 1996) himself – Malcolm Ashmore, author of the brilliant and seminal work on reflexivity *The Reflexive Thesis* (1989). This provided me with an ideal opportunity to connect my research topics reflexively, to interweave them within academic arguments for and against reflexivity, and to use the perceived problems of this approach to develop a therapeutic resolve – a form of 'textual therapy'. As we shall see, by using reflexivity, hypnosis and poetry were not only the research topics, but also informed the analysis, and reflexivity was not only the method, but also a central feature of my thesis.

Reflexivity bites by examining the analyst's position, as she works up her analytical representations. In my doctoral research, *Trance-Scripts: The Poetics of a Reflexive Guide to Hypnosis and Trance Talk*, (MacMillan, 1996), I illustrate my role as an analyst by treating the subjects of my research as interconnected, and by arguing the topics' value as analytical tools. In doing so I, the researcher, am made visible in the text, shown self-consciously arranging the objects of study in order to produce a persuasive account of my research.

Spiral reflexivity

The reflexive doctoral thesis, using new literary forms to highlight the textual construction of research and analysis, was first explored in *The Reflexive Thesis*

(Ashmore, 1989). Here the direction of reflexivity was one of 'R-circularity' (p.32). This perspective showed the ways in which the author/researcher/doctoral student's world is constituted within her textual accounts and the sense she makes of her data. Influenced by ethnomethodology (see Garfinkel, 1967; Heritage, 1984) and the sociology of scientific knowledge (SSK) (e.g. Bloor, 1976; see also Gilbert & Mulkay, 1984; Collins, 1985; Latour & Woolgar, 1986; Latour, 1987), reflexivity takes SSK's concern with the construction of knowledge, and exemplifies the way that the analyst's/author's claims are inextricably embedded in the textual forms she uses to present such knowledge.

Ashmoresque reflexivity parries attacks from fiercely protective traditionalists (still defending the ancient boundaries of the social sciences), by suggesting that the potential reach of reflexivity has yet to be fully realised. This rhetorical move implies that the future is reflexive, has many voices, and places the reflexive analyst in the vanguard of a new wave of deconstructionists. Which, of course, is a good thing.

As Ashmore's first doctoral student it fell upon me to claim the self-elected, and almost certainly fleeting, responsibility of a disciple, ritualising certain features of Ashmore's work and thus establishing the 'regulations and guidelines' for writers of reflexive theses. I did this by defining the reflexive moves of 'Mr Reflexivity' as footsteps to follow in, and consequently transforming *The Reflexive Thesis* into a reflexive thesis – the start of a new tradition. The first chapter of my doctoral thesis was presented as a 'do-it-yourself guide' to reflexivity, using Ashmore's work as a template for reflexive theses generally. My chapter took the form of six stages within six stages, to ironically reflect how discussions within SSK frequently present the constructed process of knowledge as a series of steps or stages – such as Ashmore's 'six stages' of a replication claim (1983), David Bloor's 'four key requirements' for a 'strong programme' (1976), or Harry Collins's 'seven sexes' replication of experiments (1975), and 'three stages' in the empirical programme of relativism (1985). My own 'six stages' were intended as a rhetorical device to parody a 'stages' style of presenting facts, and to show the arbitrariness of such lists of information. The six within six, paradoxically, suggests that I might have written any number of 'stages' consisting of any number of statements instead. In my 'DIY guide', I outlined:

- The six stages involved in the production of a reflexive thesis.
- The six stages of creating appropriate alternative literary forms.
- The six stages involved in forming the text as a challenge to 'standard' texts.
- The six stages necessary to display the student's knowledge of the theoretical background of reflexivity.
- The six stages needed to develop a research 'story'.
- The six stages reflecting the process of a reflexive study.

The purpose of ironically turning reflexivity into a finite number of mechanical steps that can be produced and reproduced for a DIY guide, was to highlight the inadequacy of describing reflexivity as such. This was intended to illustrate, by example, my overriding suggestion that the reader does *not as I say, but as I do* – thus the essence of the argument in my thesis lies not so much in what I write about reflexivity, but how I write it.

Taking a reflexive turn on the topic of reflexivity itself I questioned how literally the student of reflexivity should take Ashmore's notion of 'R-circularity' in writing her reflexive thesis. By extracting the underlying form of Ashmore's work, and reproducing it as a set of guidelines, I argued that a reflexive thesis need not be circular either in its argument or in its textual shape, and is, more suitably, a Reflexive Spiral.

According to Ashmore (1989, p.32) the use of reflexivity as a term in the social sciences tends 'to be subject to unsystematic variation'. Ashmore divides reflexivity into 'R-reference. R-awareness. R-circularity' (p.32), making a distinction between analysis in the social sciences being reflective because it is a study of human beings, 'merely' (p.32) being more self-aware, and the reflexive sense-making processes of members constituting their world through their words, as described by ethnomethodology. It is the latter conception of reflection that forms the basis for an Ashmoresque reflexivity. Using a relativist approach to emphasise that knowledge is socially constructed, the reflexive writer may attend to the *construction* of his own text. From an SSK perspective there is no distinction between the social scientist constituting her world in her descriptions and accounts (as analysis), and the ethnomethodologist's 'member' constantly engaged in constituting the context of her own actions.

Ethnomethodology states that a member must know the settings in which his practices operate, in order for sense to be made of his accounts (Garfinkel, 1967, p.8). Steve Woolgar has referred to this as a 'back-and-forth' (1981, p.12) process, while Ashmore takes his turn and redefines Woolgar's 'back-and-forth' description – 'I see it as more of a circular process' (1989, p.32). Both Woolgar's 'back-and-forth' movement, and Ashmore's circular returns[1] have, embedded within the metaphor, a sense of coming back to the same position over and over again.

Now (taking the opportunity for another turn, another go at Better Metaphors for Reflexivity), I see reflexivity more as a spiralling movement, with the shape of the metaphor suggesting that each turn, however lightly made, however brief, offers a shift in focus. Topics may be endlessly rehearsed, but with each rehearsal a different perspective is gained, as the text moves, not back to the beginning, but to the next turn upon the spiral of reflexivity. From my relativist position the image of the spiral has no bottom-line,[2] no realist launching ground for a gath-

---

[1] See also Pinch and Pinch (1988) for a discussion on the reflexive 'loop' and how 'SSKers' (p.181) should apply the principles of SSK to their own practices.
[2] For a discussion on the use of 'bottom-line' arguments see Barbara Hernstein Smith (1988); also Edwards *et al.* (1995).

ering of flight *into* the spiral. The imaginary fabric of the spiral turning is all there is. (I wonder, if I let it lie, how quickly the next reflexive turn would be taken. How swift would my critic be to claim that my construction of the spiral as a more 'suitable' description, makes me as objectivist – however fleetingly – as those I have just accused? Have I forestalled that by taking this turn for myself? Have I answered that by asking it? Is this yet another rhetorical question?)

Reflexivity demands that the researcher apply the principles of reflexivity to her own practice. I took this as a challenge, not only to reflect upon my own role in the research process, but also on my role as a practitioner of reflexivity. This meant deconstructing the work of influential reflexive writers, and thus taking my 'turn' on the reflexive spiral of knowledge construction.

I used the image of the spiral to return, from a number of perspectives, to hypnosis, poetry, and reflexive research. The topics became interconnected as:

- Therapy, therapeutic poetry, therapeutic reflexivity
- Hypnosis, hypnotic poetry, hypnotherapy, hypnotic reflections, hypnotic texts
- Poetry, poetic therapy, poetic reflections, poetic textual devices
- Reflexivity, reflexive therapy, reflexive poetry

and were woven together into an argument for Spiral Reflexivity. The objective was to highlight reflexivity as flexible, able to turn upon the axis of any argument, and in doing so to perform textual therapy. As with conventional therapy, the aim is to confront the complaints (symptoms) standardly generated against reflexivity, and to show that the therapeutic resolve is located in the roots of the complaint. As I shall show, in this way problems are turned upon themselves to indicate the solution.

Synthesis

The topics of my thesis, and the numerous sub-topics derived from their inter-connection, were used to demonstrate how reflexivity contributes to a broader understanding of the research process. In the first instance the central topics were linked. Most obviously, hypnosis and poetry come together in the notion that profound and healing communication arise from unconscious association more readily than from conscious awareness. An Ericksonian version of hypnotherapy, influenced by the work of Milton H. Erickson (1980),[3] academic, clinician and

---

[3] Erickson was a fellow of the American Psychiatric Association, the American Psychological Association, the American Psychopathological Association, and the American Association for the Advancement of Science. He also founded the American Society of Clinical Hypnosis in 1957, and the *American Journal of Clinical Hypnosis* in 1958 (Edmonston, 1986). 'Ericksonian Societies' have formed over the years both in Britain and North America, with advocates of his methods calling themselves Ericksonians or Ericksonian practitioners (e.g. Havens & Walters, 1989).

hypnotherapist, treats hypnosis as a therapeutic method which bypasses conscious resistance by directing metaphoric therapeutic interventions to the unconscious mind, while the patient is in trance. From an Ericksonian perspective it is the patient's interpretation of the metaphors which makes the therapy work (Zeig, 1980). Such theories of hypnosis work on a notion of individual responsiveness through a process of indirect suggestion and *inner resynthesis* (Erickson, 1980, p.38) within the client.

Poetry is frequently and purposefully ambiguous, inviting a multiplicity of readings. As with Ericksonian hypnosis, meanings are personal, individual, and derived from unconscious interpretations of the poetic (hypnotic) metaphors used to tell the poetic (therapeutic) tale. The implication that the poet is extraordinary in her ability to make sense and order from chaos through her visionary work (Eliot, 1960; Tyler, 1986), and to make a 'leap' from an ordinary frame of reference to another, more radically innovative one (Nietzsche, 1960; Brown, 1977), is a familiar image echoed in a variety of academic, philosophical and literary spheres. From this perspective it is taken for granted that poetic writing is able to offer perceptions of the world that go beyond the limitations of 'clinical positivism' (Brady, 1991, p.6). The 'interpretative soaring' that can be achieved through poetic work may 'defeat intellectual autism' (Brady, 1991) and offer a richly informative perspective as the researcher reflects upon her own subjective experience and her connection with the object of her study.

Having discussed the similarities between poetry and hypnosis in terms of responses to unconscious communication, I then explored the suggestion that poetry is hypnotic. Peter Brown (1990), for example, links hypnosis with poetry by focusing on oral cultures, with social communication treated as central in the evolutionary development of the human brain. His work traces the development of the brain over several million years, from early pre-verbal communication, through oral cultures to modern hypnotherapy, and concludes that trance is a natural part of our everyday lives. It is suggested that the human brain undergoes measurable rhythmic changes throughout a normal day, and that these are similar to the changes in brain rhythm which occur during hypnosis. These rhythmic changes have developed from times when humans relied on oral information and speakers to convey important messages effectively. Such information is retained and affects the listener in a way that Brown likens to trance. The speaker in oral cultures was required by the community to tell a story which was memorable and, as such, enchanting.

To maintain an impartial symmetry between the developing sub-topics (see Bloor, 1976, for a discussion of 'symmetry' as one of the 'four key requirements' of the 'strong programme' within the sociology of knowledge), I then made a case for the poetics of hypnosis. This was done in the form of 'letters' from Katie MacMillan, the hypnotist, to Evangeline Scribbler, the textual poet within my thesis. In response to a request from a therapy client for a hypnotic poem, MacMillan negotiates with Sleepstone over the kind of writing that might serve as a poetic trance induction (see Snyder, 1930). They conclude that a poetic trance induction is, in part, that which is argued up, and presented as such. Scribbler and MacMillan therefore produced their own hypnotic poem which formed the basis of a (taped and transcribed) therapeutic session with MacMillan's client. The words of the poem, an entire chapter of my thesis (*Spiralling Bird*, MacMillan, 1996), were spoken to the client. When he was judged to be in a state of hypnotic trance, he was then given various therapeutic suggestions appropriate to his presenting problem.

Throughout my thesis I argue a case for the use of alternative literary forms (ALFs) in research writings. In my work I use 'diaries', 'poems', 'letters', 'hypnotic inductions', 'interviews', 'plays', and, of course, formal academic form forms (FAFFs) such as this one, to demonstrate how meaning is a negotiated process.

A case for alternative literary forms

Alternative, or 'new literary forms' (Woolgar, 1983; Mulkay, 1984, 1985; Stringer, 1985; Ashmore, 1989) are reflexive textual forms which are used to highlight the construction of knowledge. The notion of a multiplicity of meanings or viewpoints is highlighted in relativist perspectives in social science research by using alternative forms of writing to suggest that an analyst's or author's claims are embedded in the textual forms she uses to present such knowledge (e.g. Mulkay 1985; Pinch & Pinch, 1988; Woolgar & Ashmore, 1988; Ashmore *et al.*, 1995). By using ALFs as an alternative to 'standard' forms the author is able to:

- Deconstruct the assumptions implicit within standard texts that there is a clear distinction between fact and fiction (see the parody/construction of the production of doctoral thesis in Ashmore, 1989).
- Self-consciously display the presence of the analyst/author within the text, and as such demonstrate the way that a writer's claims are shaped by the use of specific textual forms (Mulkay, 1991).
- Declare that multiple readings are available within a single text (Stringer 1985), inviting the reader to step into the text (Mulkay, 1985; Ashmore, 1989), and partake in the deconstruction of the authority of the author (see Barthes, 1968; Stringer, 1985; Curt, 1994 on the 'death of the Author').
- Allow a further reading, a reflexive spiralling over the last move; for example, the 'authorless text' is deconstructible as a textual device (see MacMillan, 1995), *authored* in such a way as to suggest the 'death' of the Author.

Poetry as social science

Laurel Richardson, in *Writing: A Method of Inquiry* argues against the limitations of 'supposedly exemplary qualitative studies' (1994, p.516) in social science writing, proposing that academic texts need not be as 'boring' (p.517) as they frequently turn out to be. She suggests that by experimenting with textual forms the researcher can not only invite open, multiple readings, but also gain a greater empathy with her subject's concerns in relation to herself.

However, the danger of using new and experimental literary forms *unreflexively* is that the participant's non-academic talk gets manipulated to make sense only within academic discussion. For example, in an earlier paper (1992), Richardson's own 'experimental representation', turned 36 pages of transcribed data (an interview with her participant 'Louisa May') into a three-page poem. Although her claim is as a 'sociological revolutionist', highlighting problems in sociology's standard conceptions and methods of analysis (p.136), Richardson's argument for her poem retains the tradition of social science research by being discussed unreflexively in prose.

In rewriting (and inevitably corrupting) her subject's talk, the researcher is, ironically, treating such contributions as limited, as though the participant is not able to speak for herself without the author's intervention. Furthermore, the interview is manipulated in order to make it into a topic for social science. In Richardson's case, the academic discussion is addressed to sociology, complete with authorial statements and obligatory references, while her interviewee's words are rehashed as a 'poem'. Unfortunately Richardson doesn't sustain her own argument for poetic representations. By writing her supporting discussion in prose she implies the *inadequacy* of the poem to speak for sociology. Poetry is data, a topic for analysis, not sociology in itself.

Such unreflexive attempts to recapture what standard research deletes, ironically, involves a *further* manipulation of the transcript, and a kind of 'subjectivised' distance between the interviewee talking, and the 'poetic' style of text. Subjects should have the opportunity to talk back, to have their turn, and to remind the reader that their presence is rhetorical. The difference is reflexive.

Devices such as alternative literary forms (ALFs), humour, playfulness, and irony, used reflexively, can question traditional assumptions about the research process. In a previous paper (MacMillan, 1995, p.550), I used 'alter egos' to show how the practice of 'Giving Voice' to research participants, whether by speaking for them, or by letting them speak for themselves, is itself a textual device which retains and reinforces, rather than weakens, the academic author's authority. In this discussion 'Netta Speaker', a fictional participant, criticised 'Katie Mac-Millan', a fictional doctoral student, for her analysis of a transcribed discussion of hypnosis between Netta and her friend Pam:

'In my talk, as far as I'm concerned, I was telling Pam about *my experiences* with the hypnotist, and that's what interested me – what had happened to me in that therapy session. But in MacMillan's hands all that gets packaged up and analysed *as discourse,* and recruited for a thesis on therapy talk, and on issues of empowerment. None of that is what I had in mind when I was describing my experience of hypnosis to Pam.'

Both Netta's discussion of hypnosis with Pam, and MacMillan's analysis of their talk were 'real' in as much as they took place. Speaker's criticism of this was that she was not represented in her own terms, but the analyst's. Furthermore, she argued, the analysis not only spoke *for* Speaker, it also diminished her in its representation of her as a 'victim'.

The 'alters' within my thesis, Sybil Sleepstone and Evangeline Scribbler (and to some extent Katie MacMillan), are present to question the validity of claiming single authorship of any authored piece of work. All research builds on, and uses the voices of others. The voices of the 'alters' also challenge the assumption that research questions, and analysis, can be treated as an unproblematic way of describing the research subject.

Reflexive social constructionism

For example, in a real-life meeting between myself and my PhD supervisor, I found myself present at my own analytical execution – in the uncomfortable position of being treated as a 'subject', a topic for sociological enquiry. In this meeting my identity as a poet was deconstructed by the social constructionist (in the form of Malcolm Ashmore). My response to this was to create Scribbler, as the 'fictional' poet, and Ashmole, as the 'fictional' social scientist, as the voices with which to take the next turn (and there is always another reflexive turn). In the following extract, while the sociologist treats poetry as a sociological construction, the poet experiences this more personally. By illustrating the impact of an expert, impromptu sociological deconstruction on a real person (myself), I show how analysis constructs its subject before redefining it.

Chapter Two, Act 11 (MacMillan, 1996)

Ashmole: No. What I'm talking about is the *construction* of a poetic identity. You can see the appeal, for a romantic to describe herself as a bit of a visionary – someone who should be listened to (even if she isn't), someone who has some gift that sets her apart from the rest of us. As though, one could believe, she had been selected by the gods, and is therefore different and special. Someone, in fact, whose version of the world is the best one of all, simply because she is a poet.
Scribbler: [protesting] But I don't think I construct myself as a poet, I just am. I've always written poetry, ever since I was. . . .
A: [interrupting excitedly] My point exactly! This is part of the enduring rhetoric of the Real Poet. One of the things that makes her identity all the more poetic sounding. She didn't choose to be a poet, she didn't wake up in the morning and say 'I know, I'll be a poet' and set about working out how to write the stuff. She was *born* that way! Now, what social constructionism

would say is that it is the social understanding of what it takes to be a poet that makes up the poetic identity, rather than poetic writing being a feature of some unique talent. Have you read Howard Becker's *Art Worlds*? I think I've got it here somewhere.

[The poet shakes her head and watches as the sociologist drums his index finger along the rows of paperbacks on his bookshelves. She has an unpleasant sensation that could well portend the initial stages of psychic fragmentation. At the moment, however, she thinks she has a headache.]

S: The room's a bit stuffy. Can I open the window?

A: Go ahead. Sorry, I can't find it, but the basic idea is that art and artists aren't any more unique than any other work or worker. Art, in fact, is just a job like any other. 'Genius' from this perspective is in the same ball park as 'socially defined'. Without the social recognition of the kinds of things that make a creative work extraordinary there can't be such a thing as genius.

S: But I don't write on the basis that I am extraordinary. I mean, I don't have anything to gain by being a poet. There's no financial gain. I don't publish my poems – or at least not very often. It's not a job, I just write them and then pretty much leave them be.

A: Yeah, but don't you see that being an *unpublished* poet emphasises your uniqueness. You are so different, so truly a poet set apart from others, even from published poets, that you don't even *try* to be understood. You have positioned yourself as a poet above poets, someone who is in contact with the gods rather than ordinary mortals. . . .

[A violent crash is heard as though coming from outside. The poet and the sociologist go over to the window and peer out. In the car park below everything appears to be much the same as normal. No students are screaming with fright, but wander casually in shoals, towards the building. No lecturers dash downstairs to check that their cars or pushbikes are still intact. They remain indoors discussing departmental policies and the malicious personality of the photocopying machine. No birds flock at a safe height. No one cries.]

A: I can't see anything, can you?

S: It sounded like some scaffolding falling down somewhere out of sight. Do you really think that it's a good idea to go around demystifying the mysterious, by claiming all processes are social constructions?

A: Yes I do. What's wrong with seeing that a claim of mysteriousness is a socially constructed claim rather than immovable reality? Take your presentation of yourself as a poet. . . .

S: [whimpering soundlessly] But do I present myself as a poet though? I thought I was just me, Evangeline Scribbler, who happened also to be a poet. I don't particularly seek social recognition for writing poetry, and I certainly don't long to be discovered.

A: Ah, this 'just happened' is a nice piece of rhetoric. Of course you don't want to be discovered! The very best kind of genius is someone who is ahead of his time, undiscovered and misunderstood within his own life-span, because the world was not ready for his visionary work. I mean, you're not a real genius' genius, a real *authentic* genius, unless there's a *lack* of social recognition. Let's have a look at the criteria for being a genius' genius? You need to die young, be crazy or controversial. . . .

[Scribbler lets the rest of the sociologist's talk drift past her. Her own voice has fallen, it seems, with all the other pieces of her known identity, onto the floor, lying as imaginary debris. She shifts her leg and her foot drops off. Blinks and her eye is dislodged from its socket. This image of a dismembered poet strikes her forcefully and poignantly. Has the artist been successfully dethroned? Will she now find her proper place in the socially constructed world, having been presented, at last, with an even deeper truth than the previous one. The sociologist's truth cuts chasms. Scribbler takes her leave thoughtfully, wandering from the room as though in a trance.]

While the above discussion may illustrate a strength of social constructionism, in its empirical approach to social processes in operation rather than as a piece of abstract theorising, it was also summoned in order to show the limitations within such a perspective, and to strengthen my own argument for a reflexive form of social constructionism.

Reflexive social constructionism enables us to take another turn, and to reflect upon Becker's analysis of the 'art world' as a study constituted within the 'sociology world'. In this way we can make sense of the sociologist's version of poetry as the kind of thing that a sociologist would do. Our sociologist fails to make use of the potential of social constructionism by applying it unreflexively to the construction of a poet, while ignoring the implications that this has raised for his own position as a sociologist. For example Ashmole's 'deconstruction' of the poet's rhetoric implies a 'well, you would say that wouldn't you' position,[4] which inevitably leaves the sociologist open to the same accusation. Of course he would say that poetry is part of a social process – isn't that, after all, what a sociologist, supervisor, expert on social constructionism, fresh from a lecture on the topic, would say?

Following the momentum of these 'turns', and by reflexively examining my own arguments, I am able to bring into question the extent to which poetry, as an alternative literary form (ALF), can be used as a form of analysis. Poetry, as a *topic* for analysis, maintains and reinforces the boundaries of standard sociology. Poetry, as *analysis*, can illustrate the limitations of traditional social science research.

---

[4] For an examination of the rhetoric of saying 'they would say that wouldn't they?' see Edwards and Potter (1992, pp.117–18).

Poetry as analysis

I have now (as the reader, *au fait* with reflexivity, will be quick to point out) set myself up as answerable to produce an example of poetry that can be seen to be working as analysis, while reflexively attending to the process of doing so. I did this in my doctoral thesis by being slippery. Rather than offering a reflexively 'successful' example of a social scientist doing sociology with a poem, I used Evangeline Scribbler to do sociology with a poem. Since it was a poem written by a poet, I argued, it should speak for itself, and would not need substantial amounts of academic prose and references in order to justify its existence.

Here also was an opportunity to let Scribbler speak for herself, and to respond to the sociologist's 'deconstruction' by writing the next turn, the poetic interpretation of social constructionism. The poem might be entitled *A Cautionary Tale*, or *The Social Scientist*, or *The Return of the Wild and Free* – among many other possible titles (with the title itself, as titles do, guiding the reader towards how the poem should be read). However, by being put in place both as an ALF and as a poem, there is also the invitation (which by now should go without saying) for the reader to take her turn, to make her own title (see Stringer, 1985), and have her own interpretation of the poem.

'Once there was a spinner
Spun a spire,
A circle made of steel.
Above a fire
The place he made
Met like a fist
And no rain hissed
From desperate wastes.

Flakes
Would drift from ancient faces
Fossils,
Relics from the wilder spaces
When creatures navigating a storm
Were caught by the chimneys
But would not burn.

These races were
Too weak to call out and
Too tired to return.

Each bar in every cage is measured
The thing inside is left unseen.

Once a spinner spun a hollow

Split the rafters and shook the earth
The room collapsed
And gaping chasms
Took the fire back from its hearth

In the stillness,
Now, hereafter.
Bones exhumed
Or dragged from cairns,
Displayed in halls.
Suspended cruelly,
Once in cases by the stairs,
Hit the darkness,
Fully cracked
And like wild faces
Roar and run.

Turn to the tongue.
Turn to the traces.
Unravel the web.
Unspin what is spun.

Textual therapy and the infinite regress

Reflexivity bites by revealing the researcher in the act of constructing her research world – turning her research participants into subjects, their experiences into data. ALFs highlight this process of knowledge construction, challenging it by taking another turn on the topic, and showing how it can be viewed from a different perspective. In order to display 'hypnotic' inductions, and therapeutic suggestions, and to confront the standard criticisms of reflexive research, I introduced a textual therapist, Sybil Sleepstone, to present an argument for 'therapeutic reflexivity' (MacMillan, 1996). Here, in the final twists of the spiral, reflexivity gets to be 'therapeutic' while exemplifying, in descriptions of therapeutic reflexivity, how it is constituted as such.

While the researcher does a reflexive analysis of reflexivity in order to illustrate how reflexive analyses are done, Sleepstone enters the research to address the main criticism of reflexivity – that it is an endless and fruitless pursuit of its own tale – an infinite regress, a methodological horror (see Woolgar, 1988b).

As we shall see, the intention of therapeutic reflexivity is that, as with conventional therapy, the problem can also be the inspiration for its solution. For example, by reflexively exploring the 'fear' of infinite regress, it can swiftly be realised as a figment of rhetorical imagination which haunts and harasses the traditional disciplines that shun it (ironically enough), rather than the kind of reflexive work that celebrates it. The 'infinite regress' thus exists only as a pro-jection of the theoretical circularity that restricts traditional social science. Sleepstone links reflexivity with therapy to show how textual therapy can realise, confront, and thus move beyond such neuroses. 'A bit like fairies at the bottom of your garden, or monsters under the bed,' she says, 'you have to believe in the regress for it to be true' (in MacMillan, 1996). For Sleepstone, the student of reflexivity is frequently crippled by an initial fear, stemming from dire warnings about the infinite regress. Her task, as she sees it, is to help overcome this fear, through therapeutic intervention.

One of the imagined horrors of taking another turn on the reflexive spiral is that it will suddenly start spinning,[5] with the researcher helplessly caught up in a whirlpool of analysis in which he writes about his studies of studies about studies about studies *ad infinitum* (*ad nauseam*), ending up with an analysis to which the reader shrugs and says 'so what' as he closes the pages. Furthermore, the reflexive constructionist perspective, in exposing the construction of the text, could be viewed as undermining the strength of its own position, since deconstruction can clearly be applied to itself, with the researcher's analysis deconstructing (decomposing) before the ink has dried upon the page. This *tu quoque* argument (see Ashmore, 1989) would suggest that the infinite regress is a potential problem for radical reflexivity (Cuff *et al*., 1979) and research which is concerned with the construction of knowledge and which uses its own text as the exemplifying subject.

While the fear of the infinite regress echoes an 'ideal type' researcher's concern that her research should have something lastingly interesting to say, reflexive writing has made a topic of this concern, embracing it in the shape of a monster, a 'methodological horror' (Woolgar, 1982, 1988b), and drawing it into the heart of reflexivity. This has been done in a variety of ways: for example by showing how the monster can be kept at bay (Woolgar, 1982), by avoiding getting caught up by it (Potter & Wetherell, 1987), by confronting and celebrating its existence (Ashmore, 1989), by proposing that it exists as a figment of the rhetorical imagination (MacMillan, 1996). Indeed such perspectives keep the monster alive, either by declaring it a feature of reflexive writing, or a horror to be kept under control.

A figment of rhetorical imagination

The monster of reflexivity, whether it is to be kept at bay, ignored, celebrated or banished through therapeutic intervention, is brought into existence by the

---

[5] Conversely, doing reflexivity properly in the first place might have prevented this historical fear of subjective regress. Roy Wagner (1991, p.40) suggests that had Descartes carried his philosophical reflexivity *cogito ergo sum* to its 'logical conclusion, *cogito me cogitans, ergo sum*, "I think myself thinking, therefore I am" he might have exorcised the murky demons of sub-jectivity and spared the world three hundred years of object-fetishism.'

speaker or author, and has no life outside the word or text. It is a tame, straw monster,[6] built within rhetorical accounts of how to manage it.

In the following discussion with the researcher, Katie MacMillan, Sleepstone argues that the 'monster' of reflexivity can be discussed in terms of therapy, 'revealing' it as a spectre arising from unconscious fears of the unknown. Sleepstone's technique celebrates the monster long enough to show that it is an imaginary one which may be vanquished in the turn of a page. Her therapeutic method assumes that there is a healthier textual position, in which the confidence of the writer can lead us into the realms of the unknown, creating a map of the journey there and beyond.

Entering the text

MacMillan: Can you explain what being a 'textual therapist' involves?
Sleepstone: Yeah. Um. It requires me to *enter* the text – as though it were a client's unconscious – and to reveal what is going on, in therapeutic terms. After we have uncovered the reasons for the 'pathology' [clears throat], excuse me, the roots of the textual distress, we can then proceed with the therapeutic intervention, in order to bring about the desired change.
M: And what would that change involve?
S: Desirable textual change is a resolution of conflicts. However, even as the conflicts constitute the problem, so they often also constitute the resolve.
M: Um. Sorry?
S: Well, for example, Milton Erickson, the hypnotherapist, frequently *prescribed* the client's problem (i.e. that they keep on doing what they've been doing) as a way of affecting a cure. In *Uncommon Therapy* Jay Haley (1973) quotes and discusses some of Erickson's case histories. Um, there is one in particular that springs to mind. Hang on, let's have a proper look at it.
[Sleepstone goes to bookshelf, selects a book and sits down].
S: It's about a sixteen-year-old girl who exasperates her parents with her habit of sucking her thumb [she turns the pages]. Ah! [and begins to read (p.195)] . . .
'The girl came unwillingly to the office with her parents. She was nursing her thumb noisily. I dismissed her parents and turned to face the girl. She removed her thumb sufficiently to declare she didn't like "nut doctors".'
'I replied, "And I don't like the way your parents ordered me to cure your thumbsucking. Ordering me, huh! It's your thumb and your mouth, and why in hell can't you suck it if you want to? Ordering me to cure you! The only thing I'm interested in is why, when you want to be aggressive about thumbsucking, you don't really get aggressive instead of piddling around like a baby that doesn't

---

[6] And yet, like Godzilla who returns again and yet again, this monster keeps coming back to haunt us, symbolic of our deep-seated fears, dreams and regressive nightmares.

know how to suck your thumb aggressively. What I'd like to do is to tell you how to suck your thumb aggressively enough to irk the hell out of your old man and your old lady." '

[Sleepstone closes the book and smiles].

M: And what happens?

S: After a bit of deliberate and irritating thumbsucking she starts to get involved in teenage activities. In other words, she grows up and leaves thumbsucking behind.

M: Fascinating. But where does this connect with textual therapy?

S: I'm assuming you're here to interview me on the textual therapy I recently performed on the horror of the infinite regress?

[MacMillan nods].

S: Well, just as Malcolm Ashmore (1989) recommends a fearless celebration of the monster by topicalising its presence, and Milton Erickson topicalises thumb-sucking behaviour in order to bring it under conscious control, so I topicalise the fear of the infinite regress (and prescribe imaginary regression) in order to bring about the therapeutic solution. Now there are two distinct arguments I have involving the infinite regress. One, which I will come back to later, involves circularity and traditional research. The other involves the accusations levelled at reflexivity. Think about it. The word regression has criticism constituted within it. You just have to say 'regress' and before you've said anything else, you've implied this sense of going backwards. No wonder it seems so fearful, if, as a reflexive writer you are in danger of having your work interpreted as potentially backward – not as static, not as not going anywhere, not even as a shrug-and-a-so-what kind of work. Worse. Reflexive work might actually be accused of – what is it Windy Dryden says about psychological regression in therapy? Um, 'retreating to a former developmental stage' (1984, p.31). Thus 'regress' as a word has imme-diately negative connotations, not only in common-sense terms, but also psy-chologically and therapeutically. However, and here we have the therapeutic flip side in a word, it is also a psychoanalytic technique which can be used to affect a cure. What the student needs to do, to see if his work is a 'retreat', is to do it – to go into regression. Thus, in order to be free of the crippling fear of falling into the abyss of reflexive research, the reflexive writer should take a look at the 'abyss' for himself, and see that another twist need not go backwards, nor on for ever.

M: How can students of reflexivity go into a regress that isn't there?

S: Is psychological regression *really there*? The infinite regress is neither more nor less 'there' than psychological regression. Therapeutic regression, in hypnosis, involves a reflection upon the unconscious, and a sense of journeying into the past to the beginnings of the trauma. The client does not really go back, I mean physically, into the past, does he? Well, in textual regression the student of reflexivity can examine the imaginary infinite regress in order to find out that, of course, it cannot *really* happen. Not only is it a practical impossibility (Ashmore, 1989), it exists only within the textual imagination. The cure is not so much a case of ignoring the monster – which might sound a bit like whistling in the dark – but knowing that it is brought into being *as a rhetorical device*, summoned into the argument, and then banished.

M: Just like you're doing now?

[Sleepstone nods, grinning].

M: And what was the other point you said you had to make, you know, about tradition and circularity?

S: Ah, right. Now, the other bit of this therapeutic argument is that what you see in others is a reflection upon yourself – a kind of projection. Thus, when more traditional disciplines turn to reflexivity and state that it sees nothing beyond its own navel, they are, of course, talking about themselves. The traditional social scientist is restricted to a kind of theoretical circularity by the confines of his own approach and the assumptions which form the boundaries he shall never cross. The discipline is a bit like a comfortable neurosis which will resist change at all costs. This is why there is such ferocious response to other approaches which might in some way contaminate the discipline if not repressed. Reflexivity, in some ways, is the worst threat of all, because it demands that the researcher confront her own moves and motives.

M: So the infinite regress is a feature of textual imagination, a fear of the unknown, and not so much a feature of reflexivity, as an accusation directed at reflexivity by traditional social science, which actually reflects the shape of *standard research*? Can it be all of these things at once?

S: Yes. If you like I'll tell it like a story, beginning with traditional research accusing reflexivity of circularity. This then becomes a *real* consideration by researchers using reflexivity, and by taking it seriously (see Latour and Woolgar's five-stage 'splitting and inversion model of discovery', 1986) it kind of brings it into being. This proposed danger takes the shape of the monster requiring textual attention, and finally, it becomes part of the therapy (like thumbsucking to cure thumbsucking). What therapeutic reflexivity reveals is the underlying processes of monster creation, and of course, the therapeutic resolve. Now, that aside, what I've been itching to ask you, is to what extent your doctoral thesis is going to be hypnotic. I mean, are you going to reflexively display the methods of trance induction and therapy in your text, so that your reader becomes involved in some of the alleged trance experiences…?

[At this point the discussion switches from a MacMillan interview with Sleepstone on reflexivity, to a Sleepstone interview with MacMillan on hypnotic texts.]

Having your reflexive cake and eating it

A central feature of this discussion has been to warn against turning reflexivity into a process with a defined set of rules and procedures, while at the same time illustrating how it 'works' by treating the topics under investigation as analytical tools. My own 'method' in this case was to use the research topic to guide the story of research, to create characters and events inspired by the subject matter, and to treat problems as part of the solution.

The textual poet argued a case for poetry as analysis, rather than simply as data in the research process. Evangeline Scribbler's experience under the blade of deconstruction showed how social science research works standardly to turn people into subjects. Her response illustrates how reflexivity can inform this process, can deconstruct it, and can turn it upon itself. Likewise, the textual therapist, Sybil Sleepstone, was brought in to examine the possible 'infinite regress' of reflexive research, to parody the therapeutic process, and, in doing so, to analyse research, to invite further analysis, and to challenge standard assumptions. Sleepstone illustrates the moves of therapy – therapy in action, with its embedded metaphors, unconscious suggestions, and focus on realisation and healing. Her ironic reflection and display of herself as a therapist caricatures therapy while at the same time showing how a therapeutic understanding might be used contribute to our knowledge of any topic (in this case reflexivity). This kind of alternative representation enables me to argue my case while at the same time showing how cases, in general, get argued.

This is the reflexive equivalent of having one's cake and eating it – as apt a description of reflexivity as any. By problematising 'stages' of reflexivity and relativising analysis as an 'analyst's version', I suggest that this is, in fact, no critique at all. What could be more therapeutically satisfying, after all, than to want your cake *and* to eat it too?

Summary

Within reflexivity, the suggestion of a multiplicity of readings available from a single text is never far from the surface. MacMillan has taken her turn on the reflexive spiral – Ashmole has been placed firmly in his sociology world, Scribbler has scribbled, Speaker has spoken, Sleepstone has shown us our fear of the deep. It now falls upon me as single named author of this chapter to invite the reader to make the next turn on her own (see Mulkay, 1985). Here is your opportunity, should you so wish, to deconstruct the authority of the author, and to privilege your own reading.

It is time, dear reflexivist, for the next, next turn.

References

Ashmore, M. (1983) *The Six Stages, or the Life and Opinions of a Replication Claim.* University of York. Typescript.

Ashmore, M. (1989) *The Reflexive Thesis: Wrighting Sociology of Scientific Knowledge.* University of Chicago Press, Chicago.

Ashmore, M., Myers, G. & Potter, J. (1995) Discourse, rhetoric, reflexivity: seven days in the library. In *Handbook of Science and Technology Studies* (Jasanoff, S., Markle, G., Petersen, J. & Pinch, T., eds). Sage Publications, London.

Barthes, R. (1968) *Elements of Semiology*. Hill and Wang, New York.

Becker, H.S. (1982) *Art Worlds*. University of California Press, Berkeley.

Bloor, D. (1976) *Knowledge and Social Imagery*. Routledge & Kegan Paul, London.

Brady, I. (1991) Preface. In *Anthropological Poetics* (Brady, I., ed.). Rowman & Littlefield, Savage.

Brown, P. (1990) *The Hypnotic Brain: Hypnotherapy and Social Communication*. Yale University Press, New Haven.

Brown, R.H. (1977) *A Poetic for Sociology: Towards a Logic of Discovery for the Human Sciences*. Cambridge University Press, Cambridge.

Collins, H.M. (1975) The seven sexes: a study in the sociology of a phenomenon, or the replication of experiments in physics. *Sociology*, 9(2), 205–24.

Collins, H.M. (1985) *Changing Order: Replication and Induction in Scientific Practice*. Sage Publications, London.

Cuff, E.C., Sharrock, W.W. & Francis, D.W. (1979) *Perspectives in Sociology*. Unwin Hyman, London.

Curt, B.C. (1994) *Textuality and Tectonics: Troubling Social and Psychological Science*. Open University Press, Buckingham.

Dryden, W. (1984) (ed.) *Individual Therapy in Britain*. Harper & Row, London.

Edmonston, W.E. (1986) *The Induction of Hypnosis*. John Wiley & Sons, New York.

Edwards, D. & Potter, J. (1992) *Discursive Psychology*. Sage Publications, London.

Edwards, D., Ashmore, M. & Potter, J. (1995) Death and furniture: the rhetoric, politics and theology of bottom line arguments against relativism. *History of the Human Sciences*, 8(2), 25–49.

Eliot, T.S. (1960) *The Sacred Wood: Essays on Poetry and Criticism*. Free Press, New York.

Erickson, M.H. (1980) *The Collected Papers of Milton H. Erickson on Hypnosis* (Rossi, E.L., ed.). Irvington Press, New York.

Garfinkel, H. (1967) *Studies in Ethnomethodology*. Prentice-Hall, Englewood Cliffs, NJ.

Gilbert, G.N. & Mulkay, M. (1984) *Opening Pandora's Box: A Sociological Analysis of Scientists' Discourse*. Cambridge University Press, Cambridge.

Haley, J. (1973) *Uncommon Therapy*. W.W. Norton, New York.

Havens, R.A. & Walters, C. (1989) *Hypnotherapy Scripts: A Neo-Ericksonian Approach to Persuasive Healing*. Brunner/Mazel, New York.

Heritage, J. (1984) *Garfinkel and Ethnomethodology*. Polity, Cambridge.

Latour, B. (1987) *Science in Action*. Open University Press, Milton Keynes.

Latour, B. & Woolgar, S. (1986) *Laboratory Life: The Construction of Scientific Facts*, 2nd edn. Princeton University Press, Princeton.

MacMillan, K. (1995) Giving voice: the participant takes issue. *Feminism & Psychology*, 5(4), 547–52.

MacMillan, K. (1996) *Trance-Scripts: The Poetics of a Reflexive Guide to Hypnosis and Trance Talk*. PhD thesis, Loughborough University.

Mulkay, M. (1984) The scientist talks back: a one-act play, with a moral, about replication in science and reflexivity in sociology. *Social Studies of Science*, 14, 265–82.

Mulkay, M. (1985) *The Word and the World: Explorations in the Form of Sociological Analysis*. Allen & Unwin, London.

Mulkay, M. (1991) *Sociology of Science: A Sociological Pilgrimage.* Open University Press, Milton Keynes.

Nietzsche, F. (1960) *Joyful Wisdom.* Ungar, New York.

Pinch, T. & Pinch, T. (1988) Reservations about reflexivity and new literary forms or why let the devil have all the good tunes? In *Knowledge and Reflexivity: New Frontiers in the Sociology of Science* (Woolgar, S., ed.). Sage Publications, London and Beverly Hills, CA.

Potter, J. & Wetherell, M. (1987) *Discourse and Social Psychology: Beyond Attitudes and Behaviour.* Sage Publications, London.

Richardson, L. (1992) The consequences of poetic representation: writing the other, rewriting the self. In *Investigating Subjectivity: Research on Lived Experience* (Ellis, C. & Flaherty, M.G., eds). Sage Publications, London.

Richardson, L. (1994) Writing: a method of inquiry. In *Handbook of Qualitative Research* (Denzin, N.K. & Lincoln, Y.S., eds). Sage Publications, London.

Smith, B.H. (1988) *Contingencies of Value: Alternative Perspectives for Critical Theory.* Harvard University Press, Cambridge, MA.

Snyder, E.D. (1930) *Hypnotic Poetry: A Study of Trance-inducing Technique in Certain Poems and its Literary Significance.* University of Pennsylvania Press, Philadelphia.

Stringer, P. (1985) You decide what your title is to be and [read] write to that title. In *Issues and Approaches in Personal Construct Theory* (Bannister, D., ed.). Academic Press, London.

Tyler, S.A. (1986) Post-modern ethnography: from document of the occult to occult document. In *Writing Culture: The Poetics and Politics of Ethnography* (Clifford, J. & Marcus, G.E., eds). University of California Press, Berkeley.

Wagner, R. (1991) Poetics and the recentering of anthropology. In *Anthropological Poetics* (Brady, I., ed.). Rowman & Littlefield, Savage.

Woolgar, S. (1981) Science and ethnomethodology: a prefatory statement. *International Society for the Sociology of Knowledge Newsletter*, 7(1/2), 10–15.

Woolgar, S. (1982) Laboratory studies: a comment on the state of the art. *Social Studies of Science*, **12**, 481–98.

Woolgar, S. (1983) Irony in the social studies of science. In *Science Observed: Perspectives on the Social Study of Science* (Knorr-Cetina, K.D. & Mulkay, M., eds). Sage Publications, London and Beverly Hills, CA.

Woolgar, S. (1988a) (ed.) *Knowledge and Reflexivity: New Frontiers in the Sociology of Science.* Sage Publications, London and Beverly Hills, CA.

Woolgar, S. (1988b) *Science: The Very Idea.* Ellis Horwood, Chichester.

Woolgar, S. & Ashmore, M. (1988) The next step: an introduction to the reflexive project. In *Knowledge and Reflexivity: New Frontiers in the Sociology of Science* (Woolgar, S., ed.). Sage Publications, London and Beverly Hills, CA.

Zeig, J.K. (1980) *Teaching Seminar with Milton H. Erickson, MD.* Brunner/Mazel, New York.

Index

251